W9-CDM-788

ENCYCLOPEDIA OF
FAMILY HEALTH

—— THIRD EDITION ——

ENCYCLOPEDIA OF
FAMILY HEALTH

THIRD EDITION

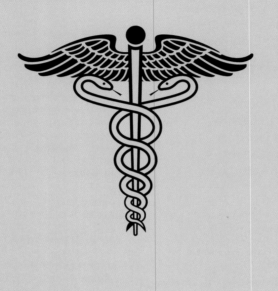

CONSULTANTS

David B. Jacoby, M.D.
Johns Hopkins School of Medicine

Robert M. Youngson, M.D.
Royal Society of Medicine

VOLUME 14

SCARLET FEVER — SORE THROAT

MARSHALL CAVENDISH
New York • London • Singapore

MEDICAL CONSULTANTS

Second Edition
David B. Jacoby, M.D.
Johns Hopkins School of Medicine
Associate Professor of Pulmonary and Critical
  Care Medicine

Third Edition
Robert M. Youngson, M.D.
Fellow of the Royal Society of Medicine
Officer of the Order of St John of Jerusalem
Diploma in Tropical Medicine and Hygiene
Fellow of the Royal College of Ophthalmologists

CONTRIBUTORS TO THIRD EDITION

David Arnot	Tom Jackson
Deborah Evans	Nathan Lepora
Leon Gray	Fiona Plowman
Joanna Griffin	Alison Tarrant
Tim Harris	Aruna Vasudevan
John Jackson	

Picture Credits
(b – bottom; t – top; r – right; l – left; c – center)

Cover: Dynamic Graphics: John Foxx & Images 4 Communication b/l, b/r; PhotoDisc: Don Farrall b/c, Keith Brofsky t/r; Photos.com: c.

Advertising Archive: 1997t/r, 1997c, 1997b; All-Sport: D Morley 1996b; Argentum: 1982; ARS: Scott Bauer 1912; Barry Richards: 1881t/r; Biophoto Associates: 1894c, 1894b, 1931r, 1932b/c, 1932b/r, 1957r, 1958t, 1974b, 2001b/r, 2010c, 2013b/l, 2013b/r; Dr G F Leedale 1939; Bruce Coleman Ltd: 1992t/r, Bill Woods 2001t/c, C B Firth 2001t/r, David Hughes 2000c; C James Webb: 1878t; Colorific: Carl Purcell 1988, David Moore 1961, John Moss 1904, 1992t/l, Linda Bartlett 1972t; Corbis: 1945, Bohemian Nomad 1989, Children's Hospital & Medical Center 1915, David Woods 2012, DiMaggio Kalish 1926, Ed Kashi 1907, Gideon Mendel 1931l, Henry Diltz 1923, Jennie Woodcock/Reflections Photolibrary 2006b, 2009t/r, Nathan Benn 1913, Philip Harvey 1929, Roy McMahon 1927; Corbis Royalty Free: 1995; Corbis Saba: Najlah Feanny 2005b; Dan Dry: 1937; Digital Vision: 1969; Dynamic Graphics: John Foxx & Images 4 Communication 1887, 1908; Eastman Dental Hospital: 2007all; Ed Bock: 1902; Flour Advisory Bureau: 1990; Garden Picture Library: 1991; Getty Images: 1934, 1935, 1942, 1943, 1946, 1947, 1950, 1952, 1958b, 1980, 1992b, 1997t/c, Alistair Berg/Vcl 1894t, Andy Bullock 1979t, Kaz Chiba 1899, Real Life 1977t, Ghislain & Marie David de Lossy 2013t; Huntleigh Healthcare Ltd: 2008; Image State: Extra Image Production 2002, Jan Tore Johansson 2003t, Michael Agliolo 2003b; Imagingbody.com: 1879t; Institute of Dermatology: 2009t/c, 2009c; Institute of Orthopaedics: 1886l; Institute of Psychiatry: Guttman Maclay Collection 1883, 1884r; Julian Nieman: 1981; Kobal Collection: 1997t/l; London Scientific Fotos: 1954; Mansell Collection: 1884l; Mary Evans Picture Library: 1986b, 1996t/l; Narcotics Education Ltd: 1999all; NHPA: Anthony Bannister 2001b/l, E Hanumantha 2001t/l; Oxford Scientific Films: Stephen Dalton 2000b; Paul Windsor: 1896; PHIL: Dr Thomas F Sellers 1955; Phil Babb: 1910, 1993, 1996t/r; PhotoDisc: Jules Frazier 1916, 1920, Keith Brofsky 1911b, 1930, 1956, Suza Scalora 1919; Photos12.com: Collection Cinema 1917; Popperfoto: Conway Maritime Museum 1897; Ray Green: 1966; Rex Features: 1925, 2006c, Andrew Hendry 2005t, Fotex Nedien Agentur GMBH 1901t, 1905, 1928, Ken McKay 1964, LHT 1898, Nils Jorgensen 1893, Paul Cooper 1979b, Phanie Agency 1976, RD/Keystone USA 1924, RIS 1906, Shannon O'Brien 1951; Richard Bryant: 1953; Robert Harding: 1914; Ron Sutherland: 1901b, 1941, 2004, 2010r; Sally & Richard Greenhill: 1970t/r, 1943b/r, 1977b; Science Photo Library: 1903t, Carlos Souto 1960, Damien Lovegrove 1880, Dr P Marazzi 1888, 1889, GJLP-CNRI 1985, John Greim 1911t, 1944, Paul Biddle & Tim Malyon 1936, Richard T Nowitz 1892, Will & Deni McIntyre 1895r, 1909; St Mary's Hospital Medical School: 1932t, 1933, 1957l; Steve Bielschowsky: 1975; T Allen Cash: 1940; Tom Belshaw: 1962; Vision International: 1948, 1970c/r, 1973t, CNRI 1895l, Paolo Koch 1972b/l; World Health Organization: 1986t, 1987; Zefa: 1903b, 1921, 1970t/c, 1972b/r.

Marshall Cavendish
99 White Plains Road
Tarrytown, NY 10591-9001

www.marshallcavendish.com

© 2005, 1998, 1991 Marshall Cavendish Corporation

Library of Congress Cataloging-in-Publication Data

Encyclopedia of family health / David B. Jacoby, Robert M. Youngson.--
3rd ed.
    p. cm.
Includes bibliographical references and index.
  ISBN 0-7614-7486-2 (set)
  ISBN 0-7614-7500-1 (vol 14)
1. Medicine, Popular--Encyclopedias. 2. Health--Encyclopedias. 1. Jacoby, David B. ll. Youngson, R. M. lll. Marshall Cavendish Corporation. IV. Title
RC81.A2E5 2004
610'.3--dc22   2003065554

Printed in China
08 07 06 05 04 5 4 3 2 1

Marshall Cavendish

Editor: Joyce Tavolacci
Editorial Director: Paul Bernabeo
Production Manager: Alan Tsai

The Brown Reference Group

Project Editor: Anne Hildyard
Editors: Jane Lanigan, Sally McFall
Designers: Jeni Child, Reg Cox, Karen Frazer
Picture Researcher: Clare Newman
Indexer: Kay Ollerenshaw
Illustrations: Samantha J. Elmhurst
Managing Editor: Tim Cooke
Art Director: Dave Goodman

CONTENTS

KEY TO COLOR CODING OF ARTICLES

HUMAN BODY

DISEASES AND OTHER DISORDERS

TREATMENTS AND CURES

PREVENTION AND DIAGNOSIS OF DISEASE

HUMAN BEHAVIOR

Scarlet fever

Once one of the most dreaded diseases of childhood, scarlet fever is now far less prevalent and its symptoms are less severe. Prompt treatment with penicillin minimizes any complications and leads to a complete cure.

Questions and Answers

In my grandfather's time, scarlet fever used to be a common cause of death among children, but now you rarely hear about it. Is this because of modern antibiotics?

Partly. Treatment of streptococcal infections, particularly sore throats, with antibiotics may make scarlet fever less likely to develop. Also, streptococcus, the organism that causes the disease, is a lot less virulent now: that is, it causes less serious symptoms. This change in the pattern of behavior of the streptococcus began at the end of the 19th century, before antibiotics were invented; nobody knows why.

Is scarlatina the same as scarlet fever?

Yes. Some doctors used the word "scarlatina" to describe mild cases of the disease because it helped to allay the fear that many people had of the illness.

My grandmother said that you could tell that a person had scarlet fever because there was a white line around the mouth. Is this true?

There is often a pale area around the mouth in an otherwise red face: doctors call this circumoral pallor. However, this sign is not specific to the disease; it is also a sign of measles, for example.

Are people who have scarlet fever isolated?

No. In the past, they were rushed off to a fever hospital, but now 24 hours of penicillin usually stops the disease from spreading.

Is there a scarlet fever vaccination?

No. There are many different strains of streptococcus, so a vaccine wouldn't necessarily protect you against the disease.

Scarlet fever is an infectious disease that is caused by a bacterium. It is characterized by a sore throat and a red, if not actually scarlet, rash (see Throat). Treatment with penicillin will prevent complications and effect a complete cure (see Penicillin).

Causes

Scarlet fever is caused by a bacterium called *Streptococcus pyogenes*. To differentiate one type of bacterium from another, medical researchers grow them separately on bacteriological plates that contain blood.

◄ Streptococcus pyogenes, *the bacterium that causes scarlet fever, is betahemolytic: it breaks down blood to leave a clear halo around its colonies.*

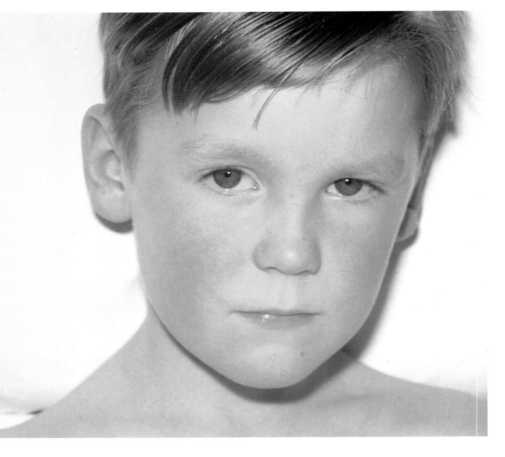

▲ *The bacterium* Streptococcus pyogenes *infects the throat, but its toxins produce symptoms throughout the body, causing rashes on the face and elsewhere on the body.*

Some types of bacterium break down the blood to leave a clear ring around the little colonies of bacteria. This phenomena is called hemolysis (blood breaking). *Streptococcus pyogenes* is a betahemolytic bacterium: that is, it breaks down blood completely, leaving a clear halo around each colony.

This halo indicates that the streptococcus must be producing and excreting a toxic substance, since the bacterium is having an effect beyond the bounds of the colony itself. In fact, it is the organism's ability to produce toxins that leads to scarlet fever, since the organism itself infects only the throat. The toxins' effects, particularly the rash, show up all over the body.

Symptoms

Scarlet fever usually starts within two to four days of incubation, although the incubation period can last between one and seven days.

One of the most characteristic aspects of the disease is that it starts in a dramatic manner, with a sudden temperature accompanied by vomiting and a sore throat. At this stage, the tonsils are infected and have a whitish crust, or exudate, on them (see Tonsils). Less serious infections do not cause vomiting, and nowadays the disease can be so mild that children do not even have a sore throat.

The day after the disease starts, the rash that gives it its name breaks out. This is a diffuse reddening of the skin caused by all the little blood vessels opening up. If someone presses down over an area of affected skin, the skin will whiten with the pressure. The rash starts on the face and then spreads down to affect the rest of the body. The farther away from the face it gets, the likelier it is to form actual spots rather than a uniform redness: these spots tend to be found on the legs and to a lesser extent on the hands. The rash usually lasts for about two or three days.

While the rash is appearing and then fading away, there are a series of changes that affect the tongue. First, there is a creamy white exudate all over it, with the tongue's little papillae pointing up through it (see Tongue). This is known as white strawberry tongue. As the exudate peels off, the tongue is left rather red and raw, with its papillae still showing prominently to make it look like a strawberry. This is called red strawberry tongue.

One of the most typical and striking effects of the disease then occurs as the rash begins to fade. The skin starts to peel off and, in more serious cases, it may peel off in great sheets (desquamation). In

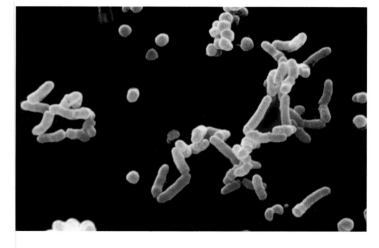

▲ *This scanning electron microscope image shows streptococci bacteria, which cause scarlet fever as well as infections such as meningitis, toxic shock syndrome, and tonsillitis.*

the past it was not uncommon to see an entire cast of a hand in the form of dead skin; nowadays such occurrences are extremely rare.

Although the disease is nearly always caught from a sore throat, there are other ways it can be communicated. It may enter the skin through a wound of some sort, and in the past it was not uncommon for infection to enter through the womb or the vagina during childbirth.

Dangers

Infection can spread to the ears, causing otitis media (see Otitis) and also to the lymph glands where it may produce a serious abscess-forming illness (see Abscess; Lymphatic System). Infection may also lodge in the nose: this is a trivial complication with few or no symptoms, but it can lead to the spread of the disease as a result of droplet infection when one of the carriers sneezes.

Other problems result when the body's immune (defense) system produces antibodies to the streptococci that attack the body's own tissue (autoimmune disease). The first is nephritis (see Kidneys and Kidney Diseases), in which the kidneys become inflamed; the second is acute rheumatic fever (see Rheumatic Fever), in which a rash, joint pains, and even heart damage may occur as a result of the body's sensitivity to the streptococcal toxins.

Treatment and outlook

Scarlet fever is treated with penicillin: this drug kills the bacteria in the throat and stops them from producing the toxin that gives rise to the disease. Even minor cases are treated this way, because after 24 hours of treatment with penicillin, the organism is no longer infectious.

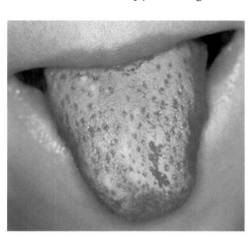

▲ *White strawberry tongue is one of the early symptoms; later the tongue turns red.*

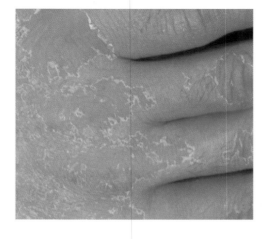

▲ *Once the rash fades, the skin on the hands will begin to peel off.*

See also: Bacteria; Infection and infectious diseases; Rashes; Sore throat; Streptococcus

Scars

I had my ears pierced two years ago, and I now have large lumps in my earlobes. Why is this, and can these lumps be removed?

This is a fairly common occurrence following ear piercing. These lumps are keloid scars, and treatment is not always very satisfactory. If the lumps are removed surgically, they tend to recur, so injections of steroids into them are usually tried.

My sister has severe scarring from her acne. I am worried that my acne will also scar. Is there anything I can do to prevent this?

Scarring from acne is a fairly frequent occurrence, with about 15 percent of patients suffering from it. It is usually seen in those who have had very severe acne that has lasted for a prolonged period. Effective early treatment, keeping up good standards of hygiene, and not picking at pimples will usually prevent scarring. However, if scars do form, a minor surgical operation called dermabrasion may be performed. The top layers of skin are rubbed away, and this leaves the skin relatively smooth.

My friend has had a face-lift, but I cannot see any scars. How is this possible?

There certainly will be scars, but by careful placement, for example in the hairline or behind the ears, they are well hidden.

I have a long, unsightly scar across my cheek that I'm really depressed about. Is there anything I can do to improve its appearance?

Yes. A scar on the face is less obvious if it lies along the skin creases and wrinkles. Plastic surgery can break the line of a long scar into smaller ones. Ideally, these will lie along wrinkle lines and, as a result, will appear less obvious.

All tissues in the body heal by the formation of scar tissue. Although scars do not often constitute a threat to health, they may be unsightly or cause distress, in which case some medical treatment may be necessary.

Wound healing is a complicated process. First, the wound is filled with a blood clot. The outermost layer of the skin then moves in from the wound margins under the clot and dries to form a scab. Blood vessels and fibrous tissue then grow in from the wound's surfaces; the tissue gradually increases, and in time a scar is formed that grows paler in color. During this healing process, contraction of the wound takes place, so that the final scar is much smaller than the original wound.

The amount of scarring depends on the extent of the damage. In a superficial wound such as a graze, there is no scarring. This is because the hair follicles and sebaceous glands are not damaged, so their lining of skin grows and forms little islands of skin that eventually join up (see Hair; Sebaceous Glands). In more severe damage, such as a third-degree burn, all the layers of skin are involved, and there may be a great deal of scarring as a result (see Healing).

Scar tissue is paler than normal skin owing to the absence of pigment-producing cells called melanocytes. There are no sweat glands or sebaceous glands, but there may be a few hairs.

Stages of scar formation
Up to the fourth week, the scar is fine, soft, not contracted, and not very strong. From the fourth to the 12th week, the scar becomes red, hard, thicker, and stronger, and tends to contract. From the 14th to the 40th week, the scar gradually softens and whitens, and tends to relax.

The rate at which and the extent to which these changes occur vary according to a number of factors. One of these is the position of the scar: hairless skin such as the red margin of the lips, palms, and soles gives rise to less conspicuous scars, whereas scars on the front of the chest, the shoulders, and upper part of the back are very marked. Facial scars also vary according to the site, with the nose, particularly near the tip, most affected.

The direction of the scar is also important. Scars are much less obvious when they lie along the skin creases and wrinkles, and more obvious when they cross joints. When the scar begins to contract, it may pull the joint into a bent position: this is called a contracture.

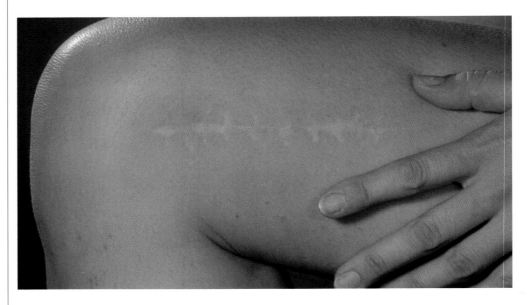

▲ *This scar was left by an operation when the woman was three years old, 30 years before the photograph was taken. With increasingly advanced postoperative care, however, permanent scarring is becoming rare.*

HOW A SCAR FORMS

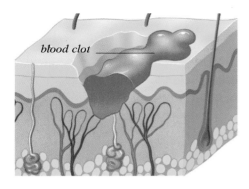

▲ First a blood clot fills the wound.

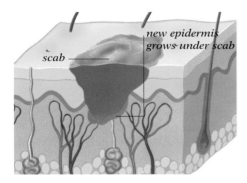

▲ New skin grows. Clot forms a scab.

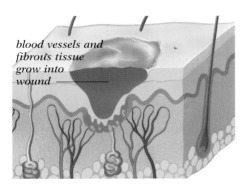

▲ Blood vessels and fibrous tissue increase and grow into wound.

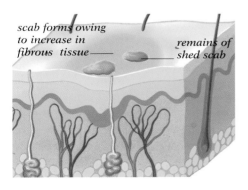

▲ Scab falls off, revealing scar tissue.

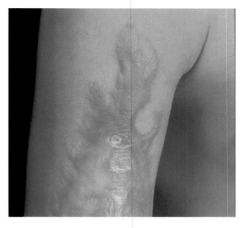

▲ Keloids are red, raised, overdeveloped scars with clawlike projections into the surrounding skin. Although itchy and tender, they are harmless.

Another factor is the age of the person. Older people with fine, wrinkled skin and children under the age of one suffer less scarring; older children tend to have heavier scar formation.

Finally, race also plays a part; for example, people with more highly pigmented skin, such as black Africans, have worse scars.

Types of scar

When a scar becomes red and thickened instead of soft and pale, it is described as being either a hypertrophic scar or a keloid. Hypertrophic scars are common among young people and are considered a normal pattern of scar formation. The intensity and duration of active scar formation is increased so that the scar becomes more red and raised than usual, and itchy (see Itches). This type of scar does not involve the surrounding normal skin and eventually disappears, but the process may take two to three years.

How to prevent scarring

Clean wounds thoroughly, since ingrained dirt or grit can result in tattooed scarring.

Never pick at pimples or scabs; this can cause more damage and also introduce infection, both of which will result in worse scarring.

With deep cuts, careful alignment by suturing (stitching) may be necessary to avoid irregular scarring.

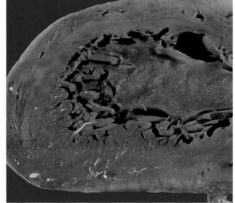

▲ After a heart attack, the affected muscles heal by forming scar tissue. This is less elastic than normal muscle, and makes the heart pump less effectively.

Keloids are grossly elevated scars that tend to spread onto the normal skin with clawlike extensions and can be very itchy and tender to touch. Keloids often get worse after a year, and may continue to do so for five to ten years; hypertrophic scars do not get any worse after six months. Keloids are rare in Caucasians.

Scars in internal organs

Scars can also occur on all the organs of the body following damage caused by either disease or injury. Organs particularly affected are the heart and brain. The heart muscle heals by scar tissue after a heart attack, and, because this is less elastic than normal heart muscle, it can lead to weakening of the heart, which then pumps less efficiently. The brain following a stroke heals by forming a scar, and this can be a cause of epilepsy.

Treatment

Normal scars continue to improve for 18 months; no surgical treatment is advised before then. Hypertrophic scars also have a tendency to improve, and steroids applied locally are usually all that is required (see Steroids). Keloids do not have a tendency to disappear and with surgery they tend to recur and be worse than before. Where scars have caused joints to contract, plastic surgery can be undertaken to lengthen the scar and allow the joint to be straightened.

See also: Acne and pimples; Keloids; Plastic and reconstructive surgery; Skin and skin diseases; Surgery; Wounds

Schizophrenia

This serious mental disorder is frequently confused with split personality, which is actually an entirely different condition. Schizophrenia encompasses a variety of unnerving symptoms, often mixed with normal behavior.

Questions and Answers

My father had schizophrenia. Does this mean that I, too, will suffer from it later in life?

Not necessarily. Although research indicates that you are more likely to exhibit schizophrenic behavior at some time in your life than you would be had your father not been schizophrenic, many factors play a part in schizophrenia.

Can repressing thoughts and actions lead to schizophrenia?

No. Repression can make a person frustrated and a little neurotic, but schizophrenia is never influenced by something the sufferer is repressing.

Can taking drugs induce schizophrenia?

As far as is known, no. However, psychological instability and drug taking do tend to go together, and sometimes it may appear that taking drugs induced the instability. In fact, this is not so. Also, amphetamines and certain other drugs can induce a state that closely resembles paranoid schizophrenia. However, when the drug action fades, so do the schizophrenic symptoms. These drugs also occasionally exacerbate the symptoms of schizophrenia if someone is predisposed to them.

Sometimes my wife shows such changes of mood that I'm sure she is developing a schizophrenic split personality. What should I do?

Schizophrenia is not split personality, although the word does mean "split mind." She may be manifesting a multiple personality, but this is so rare that plain moodiness or depression is more likely. Extreme mood changes can have many causes; you should consult a doctor, who may refer her to a psychiatrist.

Schizophrenia is one of the most serious psychiatric disorders. It may include withdrawal from reality, disorders of thought processes, abnormal behavior, and a gross inability to communicate with other people. It is the most common type of psychosis and affects up to one person in 100.

The symptoms and manifestations of schizophrenia are diverse, so much so that some clinicians prefer to talk about the schizophrenias in the plural rather than as just one condition. A variety of treatments have been fashionable but, as yet, none has been found to be universally effective. The condition can sometimes gradually disappear even without treatment; but even if schizophrenic behavior improves, it may recur at a later stage in some patients.

Symptoms

The common symptom in most forms of schizophrenia is irrational thought or behavior, which is often mixed with other behavior that is natural and reassuring. A schizophrenic patient may reply easily and courteously to questions and yet assert that his or her mind is controlled by X rays coming from the hospital radiators. In other cases, it may be a patient's emotions that are inappropriate; he or she may giggle foolishly at the sight of a person's hands, or burst into uncontrollable weeping because a window has been left open. A schizophrenic may have delusions about ordinary happenings, or he or she may have delusions of being under attack by the police, for example. Some sufferers have difficulty concentrating on television because they cannot sort out what is happening and understand the words at the same time. Others have delusions of hearing voices. All the examples so far are those of disorders of thought. Sometimes, however, there is irrational behavior; strange facial expressions, repeated gestures of a pointless and yet complex nature, flailing of limbs, and twitching. Or there will be a strange immobility called catatonia, in which the patient remains still in an unusual position, perhaps curled up in a ball, often for several hours. In certain cases, the patient will show what is called waxy flexibility, in which the limbs can be moved into any position by another person and they will retain that position. Catatonia and waxy flexibility, once common, are now rare.

The patient suffering from schizophrenia may also show unusual emotional patterns, either exhibiting inappropriate emotion (such as giggling when told that a friend has died, or flying into a rage because someone walked past his or her shadow) or none at all. The diversity of schizophrenic symptoms can make diagnosis of the condition difficult. Diagnosis is also not helped by the fact that in some cases the behavior is normal but inappropriate. This presents special difficulties when the person being examined comes from a different culture from that of his doctor. For example, in some societies it is normal for a religious person to talk out loud to God and to believe that God answers; yet the unaware clinician could easily construe this as delusional thought and hallucination, and thus as schizophrenia.

Who develops schizophrenia?

Schizophrenia can occur in anyone: young or old, male or female, rich or poor. There is nevertheless evidence to show that it runs in families. Careful research has established that this is not necessarily due solely to patterns of upbringing or to the way a schizophrenic parent behaves toward his or her offspring, but is due, in part, to genetic transmission (see Genetics).

It is very important to realize that disturbed behavior, imagined events, inappropriate emotions, and bizarre thought patterns in childhood can occur without the presence of schizophrenia or indeed of any mental disorder. Schizophrenia can occur in children, but rarely, and generally not before the child is three or four years old. It is marked by poor emotional relationships with others and the child's lack of belief in his or her own identity. For example, when a schizophrenic child is asked a question, he or she may reply as if talking about someone else. This in itself, however, would not be an indication of schizophrenia. The disease is extremely rare under the age of 15.

A child suffering from schizophrenia may show acute, excessive, and illogical anxiety, loss of speech, distortions in the way he or she sees or hears things, bizarre movements, and a determined resistance to changes of environment.

Causes

There are many theories about the causes of schizophrenia. Factors cited include genetics, chemicals, upbringing, and social pressures. The psychiatrist R. D. Laing argued that schizophrenia is not an illness; rather, it occurs as a defense against intolerable pressures produced by society. He maintained that schizophrenia is "a label for a certain sort of behavior that a person invents in order to live in an unlivable position.... He cannot make a move or make no move without being beset by contradictory pressures both internally, from himself, and externally, from those around him." Laing produced examples of patients for whom his ideas may be true. However, there is little other evidence to support the view that environment is a major cause of schizophrenia. It is probably more accurate to say that the environment may precipitate an attack in someone predisposed to schizophrenia.

Heredity

Heredity is probably the most powerful influence on the development of schizophrenia. Numerous studies indicate that the condition tends to run in families. However, it should be stressed that this is not necessarily proof that schizophrenia is hereditary, since a poor heredity and an unfavorable environment usually go together. In addition, most psychiatrists and psychologists agree that what can be inherited is a predisposition to schizophrenia. Under severe pressure a predisposed individual is more likely than others to develop the condition. The presence of schizophrenic tendencies among relatives of schizophrenics is so striking that the word "schizoid" has been coined to refer to those who actually resemble the schizophrenic in many ways but whose pathology is not severe enough to warrant the diagnosis of some form of schizophrenia. However, the hypothesis that schizophrenia is hereditary gets strong support from the fact that identical twins, who come from the same egg, show more tendency to schizophrenia than fraternal twins, who come from different eggs produced at the same time. In addition, the child of a

▼ **The Maze** *by William Kurelek is an outstanding example of schizophrenic art. The artist became so uncommunicative and withdrawn that he was hospitalized. At the age of 26 he gave expression to his despair in this painting—a view of the body seen through the floor of the skull. Once the imagery of his torment emerged onto canvas, Kurelek began to recover. Twenty years later, he painted the peaceful, evocative* **After the Maze.**

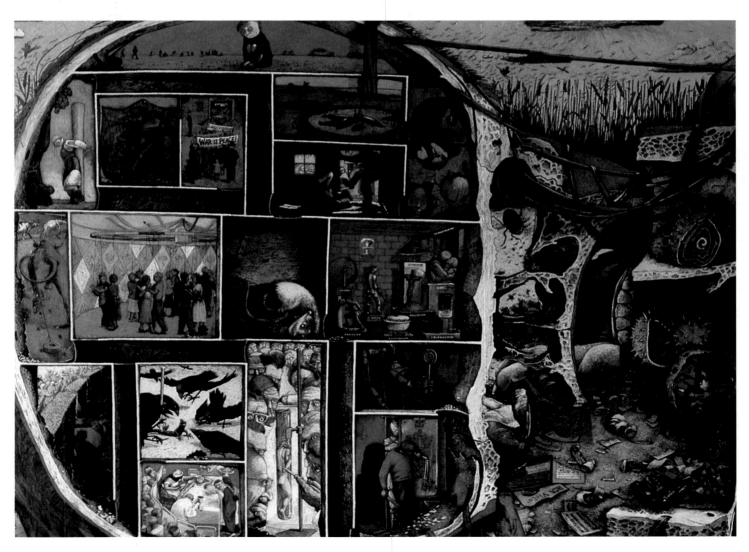

Is it true that once you suffer from schizophrenia, you will continue to have attacks throughout your life?

There is some basis for this belief, although the way the first attack occurs influences the likelihood of recurring attacks.

My son appears to have withdrawn into his own world, rarely speaking to the family. I'm worried that he might become schizophrenic. Is this likely to happen?

If he doesn't speak to anyone (not just to members of your family) then he could be exhibiting a particular form of schizophrenia. It would be a good idea to see your doctor, who may be able to sort out what is happening and decide whether your son needs help or whether he has simply withdrawn in order to work something out for himself.

Why has so little progress been made in finding a permanent cure for schizophrenia?

Schizophrenia has been recognized as a pathological condition for only about 80 years, which is not a very long time in medical terms. Mental conditions are generally harder to deal with than physical ailments, since they seldom have a simple cause or a universally applicable treatment. However, considerable advances have been made in the management of schizophrenia by the use of antipsychotic drugs and the influence of social factors. Twenty-five years ago, most patients were likely to be confined to institutions. The successful use of drugs is leading to many important insights into the biochemical causes of the illness.

Can any physical illness lead to schizophrenia?

No. External events such as physical illness or head injuries happening just before the onset of schizophrenic behavior may precipitate the disorder, but they are not direct causes.

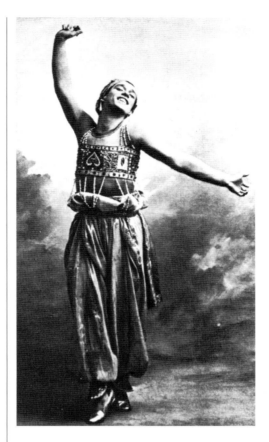

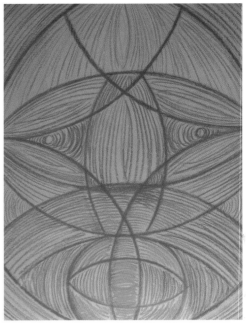

◄▲ *The spectacular career of the Russian ballet dancer Vaslav Nijinsky (left) was cut short by schizophrenia. At the height of his illness, he produced a number of brooding paintings, including the enigmatic* Mask.

schizophrenic person has about a 13 percent chance of being either schizophrenic or schizoid; if both parents are schizophrenic, the figure rises to about 35 percent.

A theory proposed over 50 years ago postulated that physical constitution may contribute to the development of schizophrenia. It was suggested that people suffering from the condition were more often slim and wiry than very muscular and plump. Research has shown this theory to have some basis: the thinner the physique, the more marked the thought disorder and the earlier the onset of the condition will be. Body chemicals are also important in schizophrenia. Research with drugs that artificially produce schizophrenic symptoms suggests that chemicals in the bodies of some people make the person more prone to develop schizophrenia. If such chemicals do exist, they have yet to be identified. There is some doubt whether it is the chemical that produces the condition or whether it is the condition that produces the chemical.

Treatment and outlook

The primary treatment for schizophrenia is drug therapy. The antipsychotic drugs currently used most include olanzipine, clozapine, risperidone, and quetiapine. These produce fewer distressing side effects than the earlier phenothiazine derivatives and are more effective in improving mental function. They block the action of the chemical neurotransmitter dopamine in the brain.

Electroconvulsive therapy (ECT) is an electric shock under anesthetic that is delivered to certain brain areas to produce a controlled brain convulsion. It is sometimes used to treat schizophrenia; however, most medical authorities are divided about the effectiveness of this treatment.

Drugs are generally prescribed for several months. As and when the symptoms abate, social and psychological treatment can begin, this may involve talk-out sessions, work therapy, social involvement practice, and occupational therapy.

It should be recognized that schizophrenia is a serious disorder, and, although many people who suffer from it will recover completely, there are others for whom recovery is only partial or even minimal. Hospital studies show that a substantial proportion of patients make a good recovery, although some may show defects in personality and a small proportion show a continuing severe defect.

See also: Electric shocks; Mental illness; Psychiatry; Psychoses

Sciatica

I get a backache while cleaning the house. Could I be suffering from sciatica?

Sciatica is the name given to the type of back pain that radiates down the back of the leg. However, slipped disks may start with pain limited to the back before the disk starts pressing on the nerves to the leg, which causes sciatica. Most people with bad backs do not have slipped disks; they have strained ligaments and muscles.

A friend of mine had repeated attacks of sciatica and had surgery that seems to have relieved the problem. Would such surgery help my recently developed sciatica?

If this is your first attack of sciatica, your doctor will probably not recommend surgery so long as he or she is fairly confident that a slipped disk is the cause (as it usually is). Most people with sciatica find that it improves if they can rest their backs properly and then resume exercise.

My doctor ordered a myelogram X ray of my back because of my bad pain. Is this because he is worried that there might be some serious cause behind it?

Probably not. Your doctor has probably ordered the test to locate the disk that is causing the pain. He or she then may seek further advice as to whether surgery would help or whether other medical treatment is more appropriate.

How can I prevent another attack of sciatica now that I have at last recovered from the first one?

The most important thing is to avoid putting your back under any strain when you lift objects or even bend down. Remember always to flex your knees when bending over.

Sharp stabbing pains down the leg and difficulties in moving can be signs of sciatica. Various treatments are available for this common condition, but rest in bed is usually all that is required.

Sciatica occurs most often as the result of slipped disks. Although this condition may affect nerves in the arms and the legs, it is the particular pressure on certain nerves on their way to the back of the leg that causes the sharp, stabbing pain that is characteristic of sciatica. The pain may come on suddenly or develop more gradually, and may be recurrent if the disks between the vertebrae do not heal properly.

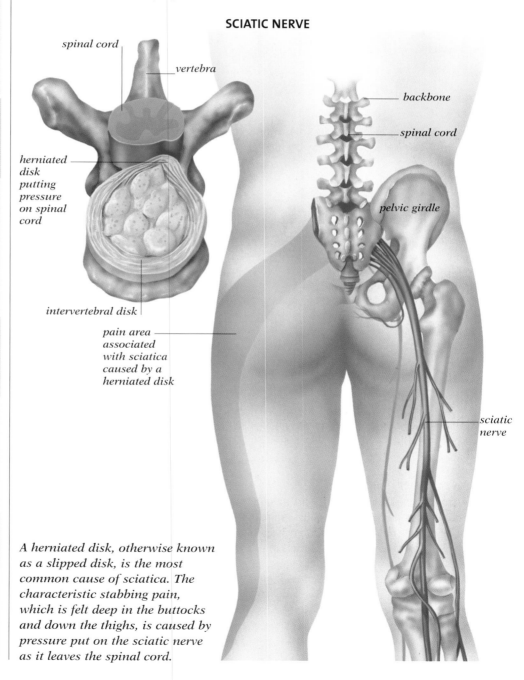

SCIATIC NERVE

spinal cord

vertebra

herniated disk putting pressure on spinal cord

intervertebral disk

pain area associated with sciatica caused by a herniated disk

backbone

spinal cord

pelvic girdle

sciatic nerve

A herniated disk, otherwise known as a slipped disk, is the most common cause of sciatica. The characteristic stabbing pain, which is felt deep in the buttocks and down the thighs, is caused by pressure put on the sciatic nerve as it leaves the spinal cord.

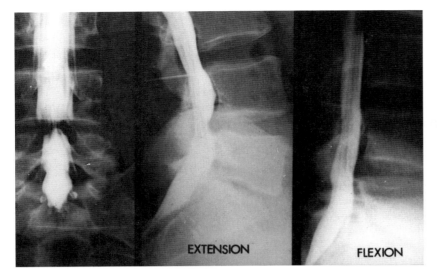

EXTENSION   FLEXION

▲ *To ascertain the cause of the sciatica and whether surgery will be necessary, a special X ray is performed using radiopaque dye. This X ray, called a myelogram (left), revealed a defect due to a protruding disk (extension) and a less noticeable blunting of the nerve roots (flexion).*

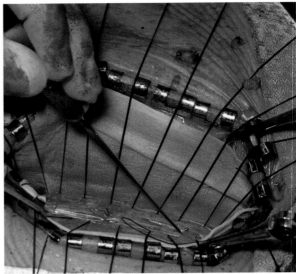

▲ *During a laminectomy—an operation to take pressure off nerves compressed by a slipped disk— a large degenerate disk is removed.*

In most people who suffer from sciatica the disks in the backbone have become weakened, either through age or as a result of excessive strain.

Causes

The disks are pads of tissue that separate the vertebrae—the cylinder-shaped bones that make up the spine (see Spinal Cord). Together, the disks and vertebrae give the spine the necessary flexibility for people to stretch and bend. Each disk consists of a soft center, which acts as a shock absorber, and a tough fibrous outer layer. With age or sometimes as a result of excessive strain being applied to the back, this outer layer weakens in parts to allow the soft center to bulge out. This condition is rather inaccurately called a slipped disk. It is this protrusion that puts pressure on the nerve to the leg and causes the pain of sciatica.

The same sort of pain can be caused by other diseases in the region of the nerve roots as they leave the spinal canal. These diseases are uncommon but have to be considered by the doctor when diagnosing sciatica. For example, the nerve roots can be irritated by pressure from a tumor in the spine (see Tumors) or from a collection of inflamed tissue, which may occur after spinal injuries or following surgery. These other causes can be identified through examination and X-ray tests.

Symptoms

Pain low in the middle of the back is often the first thing that is noticed when the disks start to bulge out or slip. This may happen suddenly during a bending or stretching action, or it may come on more gradually during days of hard work such as cleaning the house, gardening, or lifting heavy objects. As the bulging disk presses on the nerves in the spinal canal, a sharper pain is felt going down the back of the leg into the foot. This is because the nerves most often pressed upon are those that form the major component of the sciatic nerve that supplies this part of the leg and foot. Most of the pain is usually felt deep in the buttock and the back of the thigh.

If the trouble gets worse, the slightest movement, even coughing or sneezing, will bring on or intensify these pains. Sitting for any length of time, particularly in a car, will be painful because in this position the nerves being pressed upon are stretched, making the irritation worse. A doctor can test for this effect by lifting a patient's leg straight up while he or she is lying down. How far the doctor can lift the patient's leg before pain occurs indicates the severity of the irritation to the nerves.

Since any movement may cause the pain to reappear, someone with bad sciatica will only want to lie on his or her back with the knees bent to relieve the tension on the nerves to the leg. Walking may be especially difficult, with tiredness and pulling pains developing often after a short distance. Pressure on the nerve roots that causes sciatic pain can also produce other changes, some of which may be noticed by the sufferer; others may be picked up only by the doctor.

Often one or some of the reflexes in the leg becomes diminished as the nerve conducts its messages less well (see Reflexes). This condition in itself does not cause the patient any problem; it is a useful symptom because it enables a doctor to know exactly which nerve is being affected. If the pressure is severe, some weakness may occur, but this is uncommon with slipped disks. More often the sensation over the outer side of the foot may be diminished so that the skin feels slightly numb or pins and needles may be felt in this area (see Pins and Needles). This is because the nerve root involved in sciatica supplies this part of the leg.

Treatment

Sciatica due to a slipped disk, while very unpleasant on some occasions and often disabling when it occurs, will usually improve on its own if the proper measures are taken. The initial problem is to relieve the pain, and this is most easily done by resting in bed in the most comfortable position. It may be helpful to have the shoulders raised a little with pillows, which will ease the curve on the lower back, since the muscles there will have gone into some spasm in response to the pain. All unnecessary movement must be avoided.

Continuous bed rest for two weeks, with the knees and the hip joints slightly flexed and sometimes with weight traction to the

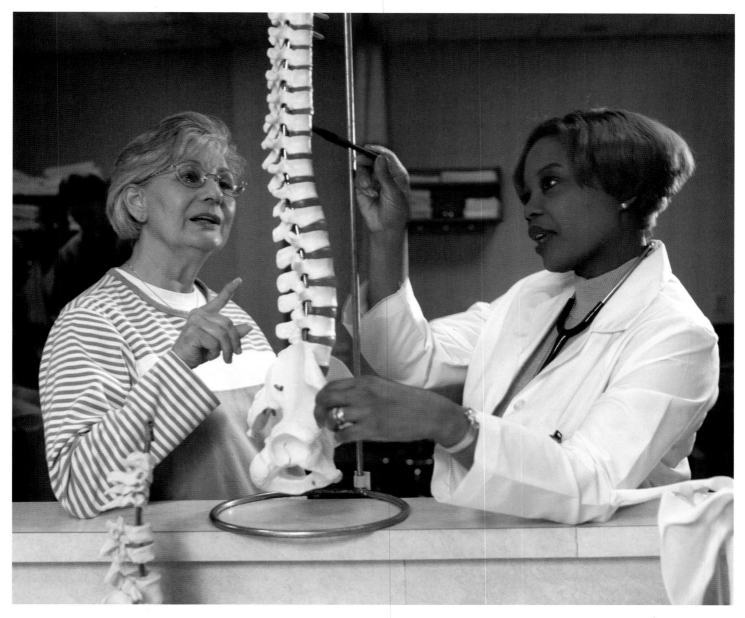

pelvis, is now the routine initial treatment for slipped disk. Such treatment will reduce the disk herniation in 90 percent of cases. If it does not, surgery may be required.

Painkillers may be prescribed if the sciatic pain is particularly bad, but ordinary analgesic drugs such as aspirin or acetaminophen are usually adequate provided enough back rest is given (see Aspirin and Analgesics; Painkillers). The crucial thing is to stay in bed and to resist the temptation to be up and about when the disk is only half healed; otherwise the whole process will return to square one. Often a hard bed is best because a soft bed encourages the spine to sag and puts more pressure on the intervertebral disks. Once the sciatica has improved, it is equally important to avoid straining the back and lifting heavy objects (see Back and Backache).

Surgical treatment of sciatica is a last resort, usually for those who have had repeated episodes that have not improved with ordinary rest in bed and for those who cannot afford to take time off work. However, surgery can be successfully performed only for certain types of disk problem, so special X rays of the spinal canal

▲ *A doctor shows a patient how a disk can slip out of place between the vertebrae of the spinal cord, which may then put pressure on certain nerves and cause sciatica.*

may need to be performed before a decision to operate can be made (see X Rays). In this test, called a myelogram, some special dye that shows up on X ray is injected via a lumbar puncture into the fluid-filled space around the nerve roots (see Lumbar Puncture). The X rays taken then show up the shadow of the spinal cord and its nerve roots, and reveal whatever is causing the symptoms. From these pictures, the doctor can see whether surgery is possible and how extensive the surgery needs to be in order to solve the problem.

If the sciatica is caused by a single disk bulging out, the protrusion can be removed. If there are many disks producing pressure on the nerves, then more extensive surgery may be needed to relieve the pressure.

> **See also:** Lower-back pain; Nervous system; Slipped disk

Scleroderma

Questions and Answers

I have the condition called Raynaud's phenomenon. Does this mean I will develop scleroderma?

Not necessarily. Raynaud's phenomenon occurs in many connective tissue disorders and also as a result of vibration trauma in people who use pneumatic drills and chainsaws. The risk that a patient with Raynaud's will develop scleroderma is less than 2 percent in women and 6 percent in men.

Can children get scleroderma, or does it only affect adults?

There is a form of scleroderma that occurs in children. It is called linear scleroderma or morphea. It is less severe than the adult variety and it does not involve any of the internal organs. Scleroderma and systemic sclerosis are most common in middle-aged women.

My grandmother has scleroderma, and her fingers are becoming curved and clawlike. Can anything be done to straighten them?

No; once the process has begun it cannot be reversed. However, if your grandmother has physical therapy on her hands it may slow down the rate of curvature.

My doctor recently told me I had scleroderma. I thought it was a skin disease, but he says it can spread to other parts of the body. What symptoms should I look out for?

It is difficult to say. In some people scleroderma is limited to the skin; in others, it does spread to the internal organs (it is then called systemic sclerosis). Symptoms of systemic sclerosis include difficulty in swallowing, shortness of breath, palpitations, high blood pressure, joint pain, stiffness, and muscle weakness. Most of these symptoms can be treated, although there is no cure for scleroderma at present.

Scleroderma is a relatively rare autoimmune disease that causes inflammation, fibrosis, and atrophy of the connective tissue. It can affect many organs and tissues in the body.

Scleroderma, also called systemic sclerosis, is an uncommon autoimmune disease (a disease in which the body's immune system attacks its own tissues) that can affect many organs and tissues in the body. It occurs in three times as many women as men.

The disorder is caused by fibrosis (formation of fibrous tissue) of connective tissue throughout the body. Collagen (a fibrous protein) is deposited in the skin and internal organs, and there is widespread involvement of the blood vessels, with small- and medium-sized arteries likely to be affected as well as arterioles and capillaries (see Arteries and Artery Disease). The changes to the blood vessels include thickening of the inner coat and fibrosis of the outer coat.

The sequential changes of inflammation, fibrosis, and atrophy are most frequent in the skin, but they can also occur in the kidneys, heart, lungs, gastrointestinal tract, and joints.

The symptoms are most likely to first appear between ages 40 and 60. In cases where the kidneys, heart, lungs, or intestines are affected, scleroderma can cause death, but many people live perfectly well with a mild form of the disease for up to 50 years.

Symptoms and signs

The number and severity of symptoms vary greatly from person to person and depend on which tissues and organs are affected. The most common symptom is Raynaud's phenomenon, which occurs in up to 90 percent of patients.

With this condition, poor blood supply causes the sufferer's fingers to become white and painful on exposure to cold. Gradually, often over a period of years, the skin becomes shiny, tight, and thickened. Eventually, the fingers may become bent into a clawlike shape, a condition called sclerodactyly. Sometimes the toes may be affected as well, but this is far less common.

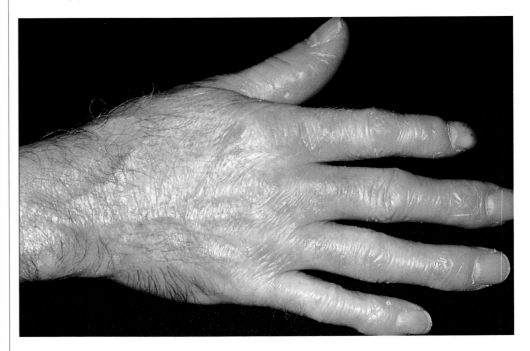

▲ *This photograph shows the red, thickened, and tough-looking skin on the hand of a 52-year-old man with scleroderma. This rare autoimmune disorder results in the persistent hardening of the body's connective tissues.*

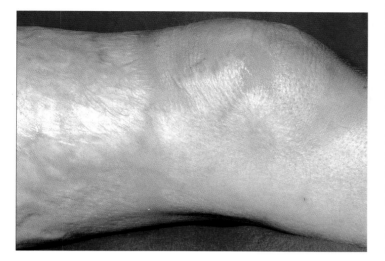

▲ *One of the external forms of scleroderma, thinned skin, is clearly visible on this patient's leg. The skin over the thigh has thin, whitish patches with pale purple edges and buff-colored margins that extend to the front of the knee. At present, there is no treatment for this disfiguring condition.*

Raynaud's phenomenon may be present for many years without any other symptoms of systemic sclerosis, including skin changes.

Skin changes will affect not only the fingers and toes, but also the face and sometimes the limbs and the trunk as well. First the affected areas become edematous (swollen) and shiny, and this is followed by thickening and tightening of the skin (see Edema). The final stage is atrophy (wasting). Changes in the color of the skin are common, and alopecia (baldness) can occur (see Baldness). Because the skin is taut, the face becomes pinched and masklike, and there may be puckering around the mouth. Many sufferers also find it difficult to open their mouths and to bend their fingers.

After the skin, the gastrointestinal tract is the most common organ to be involved, especially the esophagus. Peristalsis (wavelike muscular contractions, preceded by a wave of dilatation, that propel the food along the alimentary canal) is decreased or sometimes ceases to occur at all in the esophagus, and as a result the sufferer may find it difficult to swallow solid foods (see Alimentary Canal). He or she may also suffer from gastric acid reflux, in which acid from the stomach passes back into the esophagus, causing inflammation and a burning sensation. The small and large intestines may be affected, causing symptoms including intestinal stasis (lack of movement of the intestinal contents) and malabsorption.

The musculoskeletal system may also be involved; the tendons, muscles, and joints can all be affected. Symptoms include arthritis, which may be progressive (see Arthritis); arthralgia (pain in the joints); and muscle weakness and wasting. If the tendons are involved, there may be permanent contraction of the muscles (contractures), resulting in deformity and debility (see Muscles; Tendons).

In cases where the heart is affected, the most common problems include conduction defects, cardiomyopathy (weakness of the heart muscles), and pericarditis (inflammation of the pericardium—the smooth membranous sac that surrounds the heart), but often the patient does not have any symptoms (see Heart; Heart Disease).

The major cause of death in systemic sclerosis is kidney (renal) failure, which may develop suddenly (in which case it is described as acute) or over a long time (in which case it is described as chronic). In both acute and chronic renal disease, fibrous tissue deposited in the renal blood vessels reduces the blood supply to the kidney, leading to overproduction of a substance that causes high blood pressure (hypertension). This, in turn, leads to further damage to kidney tissue so that function gradually decreases (see Blood Pressure). In the end, the kidneys may fail completely (see Kidneys and Kidney Diseases).

The lungs may also be affected. Patients may suffer from hypertension if fibrosis causes increased pressure in the pulmonary arteries. Pleurisy and breathlessness are common and are caused by inflammation and fibrosis of the pleura (the membranes surrounding each lung and lining the chest wall) and in the spaces within the lung tissue (see Pleurisy).

Diagnosis

A physical examination is usually sufficient to confirm the diagnosis of systemic sclerosis, but a blood test and a skin biopsy may also be performed (see Biopsy). Blood tests may detect antinuclear antibodies. These are antibodies that are produced by the immune system in response to the body's own tissues, and are characteristic of autoimmune diseases.

Treatment

There is no cure for systemic scleroderma, but various types of treatment can relieve some of the symptoms and associated problems. Vasodilator drugs (drugs that widen the blood vessels, such as ACE inhibitors, calcium channel blockers, and nitrate drugs) can bring relief to patients with Raynaud's phenomenon. These patients should also be told to avoid smoking and exposure to cold.

Physical therapy may be recommended for patients with joint problems. Therapy slows the development of muscle contractures and the resultant deformity and debility (see Physical Therapy). Analgesics may be prescribed for joint pain (see Aspirin and Analgesics).

Antihypertensive drugs may be given to patients with hypertension to control their blood pressure, and thus improve their chances of survival. If a patient does not respond to antihypertensive drugs, this lack of response usually indicates that he or she has acute renal failure. This can sometimes be treated with dialysis or a kidney transplant (see Kidney Dialysis; Kidney Transplants).

Inflammation of the esophagus can be treated with antacids and drugs called H2-antagonists. If fibrosis has caused extreme narrowing of the gastroesophageal junction (between the esophagus and the stomach), the patient may require surgery or dilatation.

Outlook

There are wide variations between patients, both in the degree to which different parts of the body are involved and in the rate at which the disease progresses. In some patients, scleroderma is localized to the skin. In others, the disease progresses rapidly in the first few years, spreading to various parts of the body, then slows down or even stops.

In a small number of sufferers the degeneration is rapid and leads to death. Renal failure is the most common cause of death, but heart failure and respiratory failure are also causes. Patients in the advanced stages of the disease often require help to eat, and mouth and skin care become particularly important.

See also: **Hand; Immune system; Inflammation; Skin and skin diseases**

Scoliosis

Early recognition and careful treatment can reduce the potentially crippling effects of scoliosis—a condition characterized by curvature of the spine that can cause deformity in children and is more common in girls than in boys.

Scoliosis is the name given to a side-to-side curvature of the spine. There are two basic types. In the first, the curve is mobile (that is, it can be straightened by stretching or leaning); in the second, the curve is fixed and permanent. Scoliosis occurring in a mobile spine is called postural scoliosis. When the trouble is centered in the spine itself, the condition is called structural scoliosis, and this condition can produce serious secondary effects.

Scoliosis is described by indicating the region and direction of the convexity of the deformity. Cervical scoliosis, which may be right or left, is rare, but right or left thoracic scoliosis is very common. The lumbar region is too short to accommodate scoliosis on its own.

Postural scoliosis

The most common cause of mobile scoliosis is having one leg shorter than the other. The patient leans toward the side with the longer leg in order to keep upright, curving the spine. The scoliosis produced can be eliminated by wearing a shoe rise, or insert, on the side where the leg is shorter.

Another cause is a tilt of the pelvis, usually due to excessive tightness and shortening (contracture) of the hip muscles. Because the spine is attached to the center of the pelvis, the lower part of the spine must bend sideways when the pelvis is tilted (see Pelvis). Therefore, the upper part must twist in the opposite direction.

Another form of postural scoliosis is caused by unbalanced spasms of some of the large muscles that lie to the sides and back of the vertebrae (see Muscles). This can sometimes result from the condition commonly called a slipped disk, in which material squeezed out of the pulpy center of a disk puts pressure on the nerve roots emerging from the spinal cord (see Nervous System). This spasm is a protective response by the muscles and does not cause permanent scoliosis. It may, however, last for a considerable time if the underlying condition is not treated.

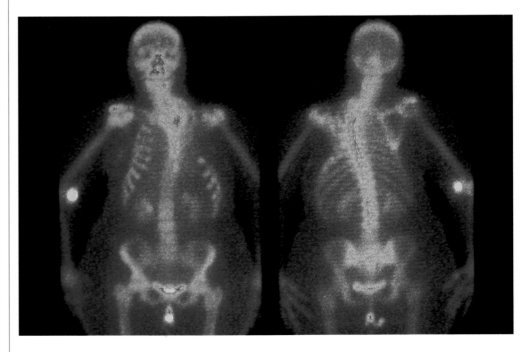

▲ *Colored whole-body scan of a patient showing scoliosis (curvature) of the upper spine. The patient is shown from the front (left) and from behind (right).*

Curvature of the spine

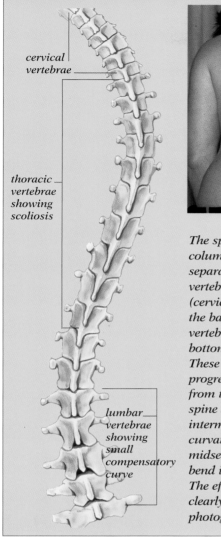

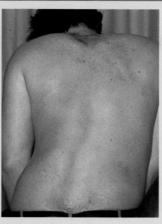

The spine, or vertebral column, consists of 24 separate bones called vertebrae: seven in the neck (cervical vertebrae), 12 in the back (thoracic vertebrae), and five at the bottom (lumbar vertebrae). These bones become progressively more massive from top to bottom. The spine shown (left) has intermediate thoracic curvature: the bend is in the midsection. There is also a bend in the lumbar region. The effects of scoliosis are clearly shown in the photograph above.

cervical vertebrae

thoracic vertebrae showing scoliosis

lumbar vertebrae showing small compensatory curve

These forms of scoliosis, which are caused by factors external to the spine itself, can easily be distinguished from the structural form of scoliosis by a simple test. When the person concerned sits down squarely, the pelvis automatically becomes level and the sideways curvature in the spine disappears (best viewed from behind the patient). When the scoliosis is due to structural changes in the spine itself, sitting does not change the visible curvature.

Structural scoliosis

Structural, or fixed, scoliosis arises in childhood and can have a variety of causes. There may be abnormalities in the shape of one or more bones of the spine at birth, or there may be a curvature caused by certain paralytic conditions such as poliomyelitis (polio), in which an imbalance of the strength of the muscles around the spine can cause it to become curved in compensation (see Poliomyelitis).

Other causes include: cerebral palsy; rare failures of muscular development (dystrophies; see Muscular Dystrophy); a genetic disorder called neurofibromatosis (von Recklinghausen's disease), in which there are multiple benign tumors of small nerves; the genetic

condition Marfan's syndrome, in which the structural protein collagen is weaker than normal (see Protein); and a form of scoliosis that starts in early infancy and may either recover spontaneously or progress to severe deformity. Such cases of structural scoliosis are always associated with actual abnormality in the bones and some rotation of the vertebrae. The deformity does not alter with changes in posture. The secondary curves that necessarily form as a result of the primary deformity will often, in time, also become fixed (see Posture).

By far the most common cause of structural scoliosis is not actual disease or abnormality of the bones or of the surrounding muscles but a condition known as idiopathic adolescent scoliosis. The word "idiopathic" simply means "of unknown origin." Some experts, however, believe that the condition is the result of unbalanced muscular development. This form of the disorder usually becomes apparent before puberty, between the ages of eight and 10, and, unless treated, continues to progress until the growth of the skeleton is complete in the early twenties (see Growth). Scoliosis appearing before or during adolescence should not, however, be assumed to be of this type. All children found to have scoliosis should be checked to ensure that none of the above-mentioned conditions is present.

Idiopathic adolescent scoliosis is five times more common in girls than in boys and tends to run in families. It is best detected by inspecting the spine from behind while the person bends forward 90 degrees with the hands clasped in the midline. The two sides of the body are then compared. If scoliosis is present, there will be an asymmetry of the ribs and the back muscles, which will appear to bulge on one side or the other. If the angle of the sideways curve to the long axis of the spine is less than 30 degrees, the outlook is excellent: about 70 percent resolve spontaneously. If it is more than 30 degrees, the outlook is less certain. In most cases, the only actual symptom is the deformity itself and even severe scoliosis is not usually painful. However, later in life arthritis can develop, giving rise to backache.

Most seriously, however, secondary curvature of the upper spine can compress the lung on one side and prevent it from expanding. This can lead to diminished lung function and poor respiratory performance. In addition, the blood vessels in the compressed lung offer increased resistance to blood flow so that the heart has to work harder to maintain the circulation through the lungs. The result may be a dangerous condition known as corpulmonale.

Treatment and outlook

Mild curves can be prevented from deteriorating by wearing a special brace, which must be worn continuously for months or even years. More severe cases require correction by special traction exercises or by wearing plaster jackets. However, most severe cases require an operation aimed at straightening out the curve and joining the bones of the spine together with a bone graft. Operations of this type result in considerable improvement in the appearance of the back and prevent the curve from getting worse again.

The principal danger of scoliosis is that it will progress to a more severe curve during the years of growth. This will cause more deformity, which not only is unattractive but may cause difficulties in walking and sitting. Thanks to modern methods of early recognition and careful treatment, severe deformity can usually be prevented. Once the child has stopped growing, the curve will not become any worse.

See also: **Back and backache; Slipped disk; Spinal cord**

Screening

Of the many ways of looking after one's health, screening is one of the most neglected. The battery of tests, checks, and examinations involved aim to spot the early signs of potentially dangerous illnesses and conditions.

To a doctor, screening means the investigation of apparently fit and healthy people to make sure that they do not have any signs of diseases that have not yet developed far enough to give rise to obvious problems. The aim of screening is to detect disease in its early presymptomatic stage, before it has had a chance to take hold in a patient. There is then a much greater chance of being able either to prevent the disease from developing any further, or to eradicate it completely from the patient's body.

To screen or not to screen

Screening people for disease when they appear to be perfectly healthy is likely to save more lives than many of the more dramatic discoveries in the history of medicine. But some people feel that doctors have more than enough to do dealing with those who are sick, without giving them extra and unnecessary work by concerning themselves with those who appear to be well. Also, it is understandably difficult for fit people to see any need to submit to a medical examination and tests when they feel perfectly well. Other people believe that it is possible to go through all the screening tests, and be told that no abnormality has been found, and still collapse and die on the way home. Certainly there is no denying that present screening procedures cannot reveal all possibilities of disease, and that there are still many conditions that cannot yet be picked up. However, there are a great many of the most serious fatal diseases that can be detected with complete reliability by screening procedures; and the list is steadily growing.

When to screen

Until about 50 years ago, most deaths occurred because no effective treatment was available for the great majority of serious illnesses. Failure to recognize a disease early made little difference to the outcome. In the 21st century, with rapid advances in medical treatment, early diagnosis is

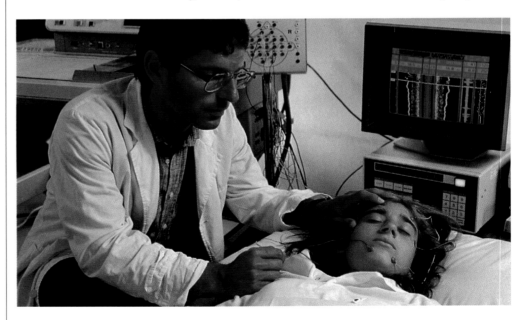

▲ *A doctor performs an electroencephalogram (EEG) examination. An EEG records the electrical activity of the brain and displays it as waveforms. Diseases such as epilepsy can be detected in this way.*

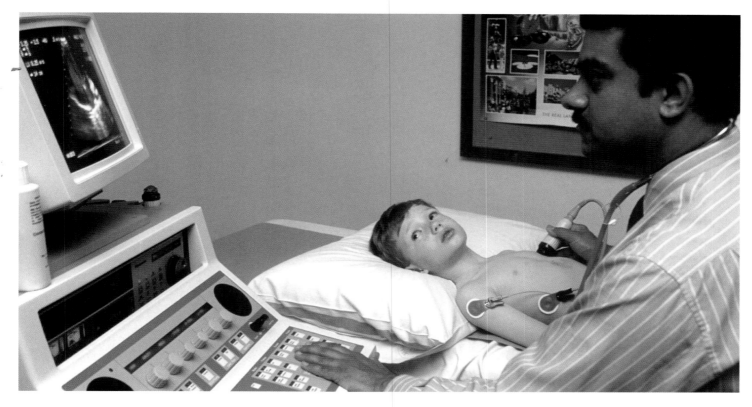

of vital importance because many treatments are effective only if applied in the first stages of the condition. Thus an increasing number of deaths, permanent disabilities, and states of chronic ill health are not due to the inability of doctors to provide cures, but rather are due to delay on the patient's part in seeking medical advice early enough. The crucial role of regular screening thus becomes clear, since it enables disease to be detected and dealt with at the earliest possible moment.

Early screening

Screening is not something that needs to be done only on reaching middle age; to be really effective it should take place regularly throughout life. A cumulative and progressive profile of a person's state of health can then be set against any personal hazards in terms of inherited, occupational, social, or personal risks as his or her life changes. By this means, the beginnings of disease can be detected by noting changes in the findings between one screening assessment and the next. Using these findings as a basis, useful health counseling can be provided that is aimed at establishing a health maintenance program designed to be effective for a person's whole lifetime. Ideally—and in many countries this ideal is now a reality—screening should start before birth. Screening at this time is concerned with detecting likely birth hazards, such as breech presentation and late development, and in ensuring that both fetus and mother have adequate and appropriate prenatal care.

Prenatal screening

During prenatal screening, the mother will be examined by an obstetrician who, as well as giving an external physical check, can call for a special examination such as ultrasound scanning. This will show whether there are twins present, or if a baby is disproportionately large in relation to the mother's pelvis, a

▲ *A young patient undergoes an ultrasound scan. Such scans are often used to determine the status of blood vessels in which blood flow may be reduced.*

situation that can cause problems at birth. Amniocentesis is a technique that is sometimes used to reveal Down syndrome as well as other chromosomal abnormalities and biochemical disorders.

Birth to 18 months

Screening at birth, or shortly afterward, detects many different types of congenital abnormality and the presence of certain inherited diseases and conditions such as phenylketonuria (see Phenylketonuria).

Immediately after birth the baby is examined to see if its breathing is satisfactory (even before the umbilical cord has been cut), and to check that all its airways are clear. Shortly after this, usually an hour or so later, the baby is given a thorough examination by a pediatrician. The baby is examined from head to toe, measured, weighed, listened to with a stethoscope, and checked for obvious abnormalities such as heart defects, a cleft palate, or nervous system faults. Another full examination is performed by the pediatrician before the baby leaves the hospital.

Approximately seven screening examinations should be carried out during the first 18 months of a child's life, largely to monitor his or her physical and mental development, and to ensure that an adequate program of protective immunization injections is carried out. Screening to ensure normal hearing and eyesight is important.

Screening at school

In the preschool and school years, from 18 months to 16 years old, there should be about six further screening medical examinations; and these, too, will be primarily concerned with ensuring that the

Is it unhealthy to spend a lot of time worrying about your health and looking for diseases and other types of conditions that may not exist?

It may sometimes seem as though all the current interest in health and screening has turned us into a nation of hypochondriacs, but the evidence of what regular health checks achieve in terms of the detection of serious unsuspected diseases, and lives saved, is too impressive and important to ignore. After screening, you know that everything has been done to make sure your body is healthy and—if the results are favorable—you can relax for another year, without the constant anxiety of not knowing what sort of state your health is in and worrying that something might be about to go dangerously wrong. It is not suggested that people should be thinking constantly about their state of health, or having it screened every few weeks. A regular check, perhaps once a year, is all that is required. After all, you would have a piece of machinery regularly serviced.

Are screening examinations expensive?

Screening is unavoidably expensive because it is very time-consuming for the doctors, nurses, laboratory, and X-ray staff to perform; and expensive materials and equipment may be involved. Look at your health insurance and see if you are covered for this type of examination. You could ask your doctor for an examination, but you must expect to pay a fee for it. However, this arrangement would have the advantage that, because your doctor has personal knowledge of your background and the circumstances of your life, his or her assessment and advice could be much more worthwhile than that of a doctor who is not familiar with you. Being screened does not mean that you are necessarily healthy; keep an eye on your health between screenings.

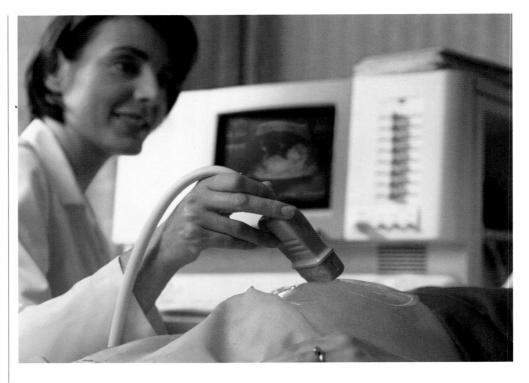

▲ *Ultrasound scanning uses high-frequency sound waves to look at the movement of a fetus and to monitor fetal growth.*

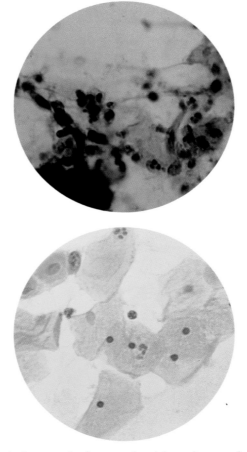

▲ *One cervical smear (top) has abnormal cells; the other (bottom) is normal.*

patient's physical development and mental development are taking place at a normal rate. Any abnormalities that are detected can then be fully investigated and treated. Special attention is paid to any changes or abnormalities in height, weight, vision, and hearing. Also, children will be observed for signs of poor nutrition, neglect, and even maltreatment. As far as possible the doctor will try to assess a child's intellectual development during the course of the examination.

It is after the school years that the regular screening of a person often breaks down. Screening tests at regular intervals should be as valuable as they were earlier in life, but usually, unless they occur in the course of a person's employment, they are likely not to happen at all.

It is important, therefore, that people who are not offered regular health screening in any other way should make the effort to organize it for themselves. The results can be well worth the time and money involved.

The ideal person to carry out a health screening is someone's own personal physician, since he or she will have the most detailed and intimate knowledge of a patient's medical history, personality, occupation, and family situation. He or she is also the most appropriate person to put the findings into the right perspective, and to give

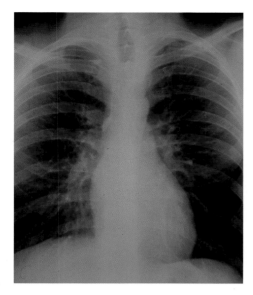

▲ *A chest X ray can reveal if there are any potential problems in the lungs: this one is clear.*

advice geared to the patient's personal circumstances. In the United States whether or not health insurance covers such routine screening examinations depends on which health plan someone has. Nevertheless many doctors are willing to carry out screening examinations.

What happens at a screening

The screening process or consultation consists of three separate stages. The first part, often conducted as a questionnaire, is designed to obtain as much information about the patient's past and present health, personal circumstances, and state of mind as he or she is able to supply. As well as details of age, occupation, habits, and personal life, a patient would be asked about any current symptoms of illness, and feelings about his or her social, sexual, home, and working life.

The second stage consists of a full physical examination, and special investigations such as blood tests, X rays, urine tests, and electrocardiogram. The physical examination will usually take between 30 and 60 minutes. The doctor will check for any abnormalities, such as spots, rashes, lumps, and swellings, and will look for any internal swelling or for areas that are particularly tender. The doctor will carefully check many of the bodily functions, for these can reveal the early stages of many diseases. Of special interest are weight, height, and blood pressure. Blood tests can reveal conditions such as anemia, liver disease, gout, and kidney problems. A urine test can show up evidence of diabetes and of some urinary diseases.

The final, and in many ways the most important, stage will probably not take place until a week or more after the initial physical examination, since it is likely to take time to assemble the results of the tests done so far. The doctor will go through the results of the

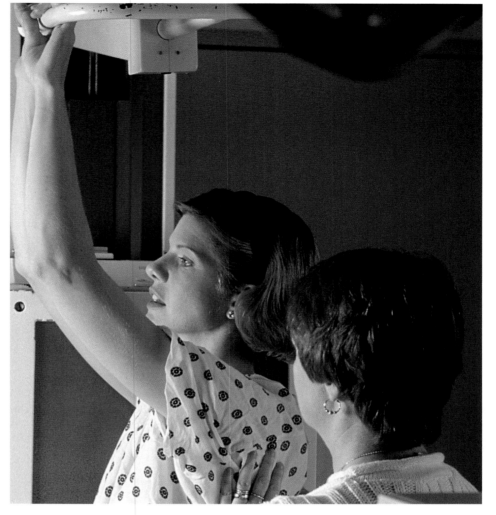

▲ *This woman is about to undergo a routine mammogram to screen for any abnormalities in the breast tissue. Regular self-examination of breasts can detect lumps that might require further investigation.*

screening with the patient and pick out any findings that could indicate potential trouble ahead. He or she will advise the patient what should be done either immediately or in the future to deal with the situation.

Other types of screening

Other types of screening that are more readily available include dental examinations and vision tests. Special treatment clinics will also give a complete examination for sexually transmitted diseases without a patient's needing to be referred to the clinic by a physician (see Sexually Transmitted Diseases).

Well-woman clinics

Female patients can be referred to a well-woman clinic where they can have a physical examination, and also a vaginal and breast check. Self-monitoring is valuable; women can examine their breasts and notice changes in bodily functions, especially weight.

See also: Amniocentesis; Breasts; Risk analysis

Scurvy

Is it true that bottle-fed babies are more at risk of developing scurvy than breast-fed babies?

Cow's milk contains very little vitamin C, although this vitamin is added to most powdered formulas. However, juices that contain a lot of vitamin C are often given to very young infants. A breast-fed baby is at risk of developing scurvy only if his or her mother also has it.

Is scurvy a very painful condition?

If the teeth are still present in the mouth, it can be very painful. The pain of scurvy is most striking in babies. The disease causes bleeding into the periosteum, the fibrous covering of the bones, and this is so painful that the baby may adopt a characteristic froglike posture.

Can scurvy be prevented if fresh fruit and vegetables containing vitamin C aren't available?

Yes, there are a number of ways of getting the vitamin apart from the normal sources such as citrus fruits. Seaweed and rose hips contain a large amount. The other likely source is in germinating seeds, such as mustard and cress.

I understand that scurvy causes the teeth to fall out, but what happens if I have already lost all my teeth?

One of the main effects of scurvy is on the teeth and gums, which bleed and become infected, but if you have already lost your teeth, your gums will not be affected.

Is there vitamin C in a food like potatoes?

Yes, but the amount varies according to how long they have been stored. New potatoes contain more. Also, prolonged cooking will destroy the vitamin.

This disease was once very common, especially among sailors. The value of fresh fruit and other sources of vitamin C in the diet has been recognized, and scurvy has now almost disappeared.

Scurvy was once such a common disease that it found its way into the English language as a term of abuse. Like all diseases of inadequate nutrition, it is now rare in Western countries, although it certainly still occurs. There are many people with a diet that is deficient, and they may find themselves on the borderline of developing scurvy (see Diet).

Scurvy results from a deficiency of vitamin C, which is found mainly in fresh fruit and vegetables. Although it was once very common, the disease attracted most attention at sea. It was recognized that sailors making long voyages were likely to suffer from scurvy and that English sailors in particular were prone to attack: fresh fruit, like oranges and lemons, which are a very good source of the vitamin, were not a staple in the English diet.

By the early part of the 18th century, people were beginning to realize that fruit might be of value in warding off the disease. In 1747, the British naval ship HMS *Salisbury* set sail across the Atlantic. During the voyage, James Lind, the ship's surgeon, proved that fresh fruit prevented the disease. In a controlled trial, he gave 12 sailors with scurvy some of the fruit, while others were given popular cures of the time such as seawater or nutmeg. Only those who ate the fresh fruit were cured.

The concept of a controlled trial is the basis of nearly all drug research today, and Lind was the first man to use this approach in any disease. Despite this magnificent piece of scientific demonstration, it still took the Royal Navy about 40 years to make fruit issue standard on long voyages. The regulated administration of lime juice from 1865 onward prompted people to nickname English sailors "limeys."

Symptoms

Vitamin C is essential for the formation of the normal form of the protein collagen (see Protein). This is one of the principal building materials of the body. Collagen is involved in most of the connective tissues, in the walls of the arteries (see Arteries and Artery Disease), in the formation of the gums and the fibers that hold the teeth in place, and in the main part of the bones.

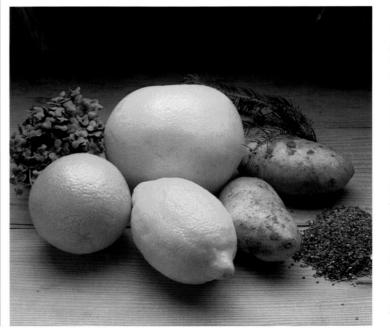

◄ *Citrus fruits, such as lemons, grapefruit, and oranges, are a well-known source of vitamin C, but other sources are less well known, such as potatoes and mustard and cress. All these foods will help prevent scurvy. However, the vitamin C content of these foods will be decreased if they are overcooked or stored for long periods of time.*

Without adequate vitamin C, much of the structural tissue of the body is weakened, bleeding occurs easily in any part that is exposed to trauma, and the teeth become loose and may fall out. Most of the other symptoms of the disease are related to abnormal bleeding. In adults this tends to affect the skin and the gums, although the gums are involved only in people who still have their own teeth. In the early stages of the disease there is bleeding from around the base of the teeth. After this the gums retract from the teeth, and eventually the teeth will fall out (see Gums and Gum Diseases; Teeth and Teething).

In the skin, the bleeding usually takes the form of large bruises that tend to occur in the thigh area of the legs (see Bruises). However, the areas of bleeding may be much smaller and are generally concentrated around the legs; sometimes there are little red hemorrhages visible around the roots of body hairs.

As the disease progresses, bleeding may occur in deeper tissues such as the muscles or the intestines and stomach. As well as causing bleeding, scurvy also seems to interfere with the formation of blood cells, resulting in a form of anemia in the sufferer (see Anemia).

Vitamin C is essential for the skin to heal properly, and another characteristic of scurvy is that wounds may not heal.

Who is at risk?

In countries like the United States, scurvy is very uncommon and it almost always affects either the elderly or those whose social isolation leads to a deficient diet. It is rare in children and infants. In the past, children who were bottle-fed were more likely to be affected: this is because cow's milk contains almost no vitamin C.

Although the disease does occur in elderly women on inadequate diets, in the United States it seems to affect men in particular. The typical sufferer from scurvy these days is a bachelor living alone who smokes heavily. It is not clear why smoking seems to put some people at risk, but there does seem to be an association (see Smoking).

Treatment

The treatment is simple: give vitamin C by mouth. Improvement will be immediate and will continue over the course of a few weeks. It is obviously important to look for signs of other vitamin deficiencies (see Vitamins) and in practice most doctors will prescribe a mixture of vitamins.

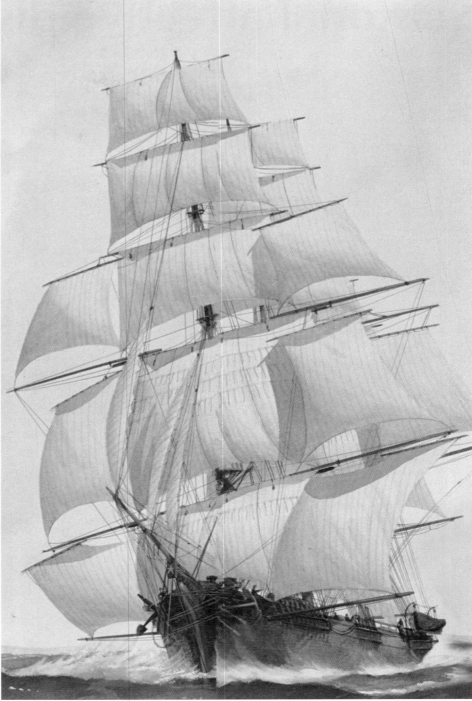

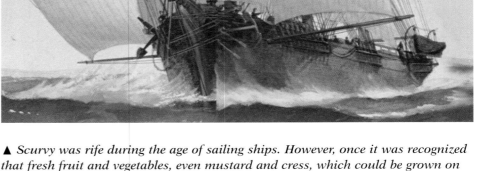

▲ *Scurvy was rife during the age of sailing ships. However, once it was recognized that fresh fruit and vegetables, even mustard and cress, which could be grown on board ship, prevented the disease, scurvy in sailors ceased.*

Once the disease has been treated, prevention relies on making sure that the affected patient keeps to a normal diet. This can be difficult, since there is nearly always some degree of social isolation involved for the patient to get the disease in the first place.

See also: Bones; Hemorrhage; Nutrition; Vitamin C

Seasonal affective disorder

Doctors have long argued about the reality of a disorder in which mood is affected by the season. However, recent research has tended to increasingly support the existence of seasonal affective disorder (SAD).

Questions and Answers

My psychiatrist says that I am suffering from SAD and that I need light therapy. What does light therapy involve, and are there any serious side effects?

Light therapy, or phototherapy, simply involves the exposure of the face to light of fairly high intensity, usually for less than an hour a day. You can sit up and read a book while undergoing the treatment. Research suggests that to be most effective, light therapy should be given in the early morning so as to shift the phase of the secretion of melatonin by the pineal gland.

Does light therapy really cure SAD?

It is hard to say for certain. By its nature, this is not the type of treatment that can be properly tested in a controlled manner. Few psychiatrists would rely on this therapy alone in cases of severe seasonal depression.

Is there a connection between SAD and premenstrual syndrome (PMS)?

There is no direct connection. The two states share certain symptoms, such as depression and irritability, but that is true of many conditions. There is, however, some evidence that women who are more affected by PMS in winter than in summer may be helped by light therapy.

I read that SAD has to do with the melatonin produced by the pineal gland under the influence of light and dark. Can you explain this?

The supposition is that sufferers from SAD produce higher levels of melatonin because the pineal gland is being overstimulated through the eyes and the sympathetic nerves. However, the truth is that the pineal gland produces melatonin only in the dark. Light in the eyes actually inhibits melatonin production.

Seasonal affective disorder (SAD) is a condition of mild to severe depression brought on by winter. Strictly, the term "affect" means the emotional feeling, tone, and mood attached to a thought, and the external manifestations of that feeling. The term is, however, often used in a looser sense to refer simply to mood.

One problem doctors have with SAD is that nearly everyone experiences mood changes as a result of weather changes. It is almost universal to feel a degree of elation in bright, sunny weather and depressed in dull, rainy weather. This being so, it is questionable whether such reactions should be described as a disorder.

Historical perspective

There is nothing new in the recognition of the link between depression and the onset of winter. The word "gloom" is used to describe both an environmental state and a feeling. This link has been noted especially in Arctic and Antarctic areas, in which winter nights are long and dark. In 1898, the Arctic explorer Frederick Cook recorded in his journal: "The curtain of blackness which has fallen over the outer world of icy desolation has also descended upon the inner world of our souls." All members of the expedition were thoroughly depressed. The doctor on Robert Peary's Arctic expedition also recorded similar reactions, not only in the members of the expedition but also in the Inuit people that they encountered. The critical factor appears to be the length of daylight, which is, of course, related to the latitude. People living near the equator, where the days and nights are of relatively unchanging length, are much less affected in this way.

It has also been known for a long time that there is a strong seasonality in mortality, especially among older people. Most of these deaths are due to the thickening of the blood (hemoconcentration) that results from exposure to cold; a very few are the result of

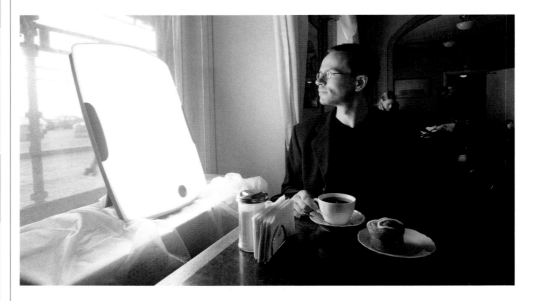

▲ *This cafe in Helsinki, Finland, provides special lamps that simulate artificial daylight to keep customers from falling victim to seasonal affective disorder (SAD) during the long winter days that are common in Arctic regions. The disease may affect as many as one in 20 people. Many doctors, however, are not convinced that an actual disorder exists. They believe that feeling depressed in winter is simply a part of human existence.*

hypothermia. However, because mortality is also related to state of mind, some of the deaths may be due to winter depression.

It is also known that there is a category of major clinical depression in which the onset is three times as common in the 60-day period between the beginning of October and the end of November than in the rest of the year. Clinical depression is associated with a high incidence of suicide, but also with a raised incidence of deaths from nonvoluntary causes (see Depression).

Does SAD exist?

Medical opinion seems to be beginning to support SAD as a genuine clinical entity. However, the Diagnostic and Statistical Manual of Mental Disorders of the American Psychiatric Association (DSM-IV) refers only to seasonal depression and seasonal mood disorders rather than to a specific psychiatric condition (see Psychiatry). For this reason its main features remain ill-defined. Popular accounts of seasonal affective disorder, and its memorable acronym, have led many people outside the medical profession to conclude, wrongly, that it is abnormal to feel depressed in wintertime.

This view has been strengthened by a number of research projects into the prevalence of SAD in different latitudes in the United States. One such project, based on a 15-point questionnaire completed by large numbers of randomly selected subjects, reported that the prevalence varied strongly with latitude, being higher in the more northerly states. The reported figures were remarkable. In some northern states, such as Minnesota, prevalence was said to be as high as one person in 100; while in some southern states, such as Florida, the prevalence was as low as one person in over 16,000. There were, however, some notable anomalies. Idaho in the north had very low figures; Arkansas in the south had high figures. These suggest that factors other than length of daylight may have been operating.

Those who believe in SAD assert that it is characterized by a strong tendency to excessive sleep (hypersomnia, a symptom that is not characteristic of depression) and a craving for carbohydrates that often results in excessive weight gain. Most of the excess weight is, however, lost when the condition passes with the onset of spring. There are also less specific effects such as fatigue, loss of energy, and a reduction in the desire for social activity (see Fatigue). Perhaps significantly, some research projects have shown that it was only people who had heard of SAD who claimed to suffer seasonal shifts in mood.

SAD research

The most interesting aspects of SAD research relate to the link between light and hormonal changes (see Hormones). The pineal gland is a tiny, solid, midline organ buried deep in the brain (see Glands). For many years its function was unknown. The 18th-century French philosopher René Descartes believed that it was the seat of the soul. It is now known that the pineal gland receives nerve fibers from the automatic part of the nervous system, the autonomic nervous system, and secretes a hormone called melatonin (see Autonomic Nervous System). Melatonin, which was discovered in 1858, is secreted almost entirely at night, so it was natural for researchers to suppose that the higher levels of this hormone caused the depression, and that people with SAD might be producing undue amounts of melatonin. However, when people with SAD are studied it is found that their melatonin production and responses to the rhythm of day and night are exactly the same as those of anyone else.

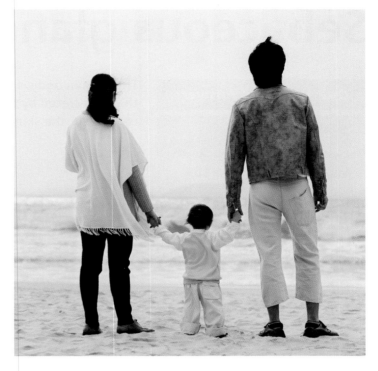

▲ *Even in warmer climates, a series of overcast days may lead people to feel down or depressed.*

A research project studied the prevalence of putative seasonal affective disorder among people in the Interlake district of Manitoba, Canada, who are wholly descended from Icelandic emigrants, and compared them with populations along the East Coast of the United States. This study found, unexpectedly, that the rates were nearly three times higher in the United States than in Canada. A study conducted in Iceland gave a similarly surprising result.

Obviously, the relationship between the prevalence of seasonal affective disorder and geographic latitude is much more complex than had previously been thought.

Treatment of SAD

If SAD is caused by insufficient light, then it should respond to light exposure. A number of trials have been done and they seem to have had some worthwhile effect. The trials have, however, been criticized. Trials of the efficacy of a treatment should always include placebo controls that are known to be ineffective (see Placebo Effect). Also, the subjects and the researchers should be unaware, until the trial is over, of which patients are having the real treatment and which the placebo. These criteria are impossible with light treatment. In addition, intense light can increase the risk of skin cancer (see Skin and Skin Diseases).

Bright light therapy given in the early morning will inhibit melatonin production and advance the phase of the circadian rhythm driven by melatonin. The neurotransmitter serotonin is a precursor of melatonin and it is possible that by producing less melatonin, serotonin levels may be raised. Antidepressant drugs such as Prozac work by raising the serotonin levels in the brain (see Psychotropic Drugs).

See also: **Insomnia; Melatonin; Moods**

Sebaceous glands

The human body is covered with a thin film of sebum, a greasy substance that is secreted by the sebaceous glands. The glands act as a protective coating for the skin and the hair.

Questions and Answers

My skin is greasy; is something wrong with my sebaceous glands?

Sebaceous glands are built into the skin to produce a protective layer of grease over the skin. Many people think something is wrong if their skin looks oily, even though grease is normal. The amount of grease on people's skin varies throughout the population, but is largely controlled by hormones and genetic predisposition and is not an abnormality of the actual glands.

Does diet influence sebum production or greasiness?

For years researchers have tried to connect fat intake in the diet with sebum production but no connection has been shown. In other words there really is no connection between eating junk food and having greasy skin.

Does the Pill alter the activity of sebaceous glands?

Sebaceous gland secretions are controlled by hormones. Male hormones, such as testosterone, switch the glands on; the female hormone estrogen switches them off. For this reason, a pill containing estrogen has been used to reduce sebaceous gland activity and to treat acne. The progesterone in the Pill works the opposite way and may increase gland activity. The result depends on which hormone in the Pill the user responds to most. The Pill can make skin more greasy, or it can make skin drier.

What exactly is a sebaceous cyst?

When a sebaceous gland is blocked by dirt or hard wax, the production of sebum continues but sebum cannot escape, causing the gland to swell and to become a sebaceous cyst.

Sebaceous glands are tiny glands in the skin that are found all over the body except for the palms of the hands and the soles of the feet. Although often associated with hair follicles, they also occur independently, over the nose, forehead, center of the back, and chest.

Sebaceous glands are so called because they produce a greasy substance called sebum, which is a mixture of water, fats, waxes, and cholesterol. It is produced as a result of cells dying within the gland and is secreted through hair follicles. Sebum covers the skin with a greasy film.

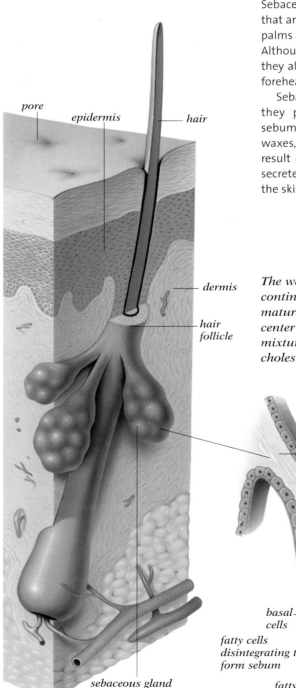

pore
epidermis
hair
dermis
hair follicle
sebaceous gland

SEBUM PRODUCTION

The wall of each sebaceous gland is continually producing new cells. As they mature, they are pushed toward the center and then dissolve into sebum—a mixture of water, fats, waxes, and cholesterol.

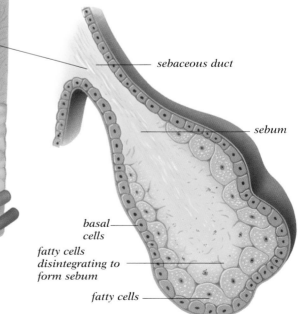

sebaceous duct
sebum
basal cells
fatty cells disintegrating to form sebum
fatty cells

Functions

Sebaceous glands produce sebum, which has two important roles to play. First, it provides a waterproof layer to protect the skin (see Skin and Skin Diseases). This works in two ways: in warm dry climates it helps to retain moisture and stops the skin from getting too dry; then, if the skin is submerged in water, sebum prevents overhydration and protects the skin by a waterproofing function.

Second, sebum appears to protect the skin against infection. Bacteria and fungi that might otherwise grow on the skin seem to be inhibited by substances in sebum. This is why people who are continually removing sebum—for example, when using detergents without protecting the hands with rubber gloves—seem to be particularly at risk of skin infections. Similarly, removing the sebum layer by repeatedly cleansing the skin with alcohol quickly leads to dry skin which can become infected.

How sebum is produced

Sebum production is controlled by hormones (see Hormones), in particular the sex hormones. Children, therefore, tend to produce relatively little sebum until they reach puberty, at which time production increases by as much as fivefold.

The male sex hormone, testosterone, seems to play an important part in sebaceous gland activity, and, as a result, men tend to produce slightly more sebum than do women. In women, sebum production is stimulated by male hormones made by the adrenal glands. The amount produced, however, is further controlled by the activity of the female sex hormones. Estrogen diminishes sebaceous gland activity, while progesterone encourages it. The fluctuation of these hormones during the female menstrual cycle accounts for changes in the greasiness of some women's skin. Other hormones are also important in promoting sebum production. Thyroid and pituitary hormones all influence secretion, and growth hormones seem to have a special controlling role.

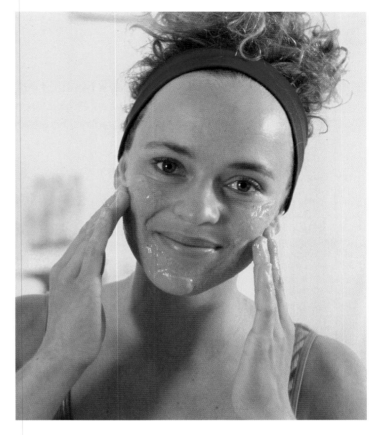

▲ *Avoiding harsh soaps and applying moisturizing creams regularly is the best way to keep very dry skin supple.*

Everyone's skin has sebaceous glands, which all produce sebum. Some people, however, find that their skin is excessively greasy, while others have very dry skin.

Excessive greasiness is particularly common during adolescence, when sebaceous glands may be rather overactive. It is a condition that is often inherited and will usually clear in time. Meanwhile, people who have greasy skin will find that the best way to deal with the problem is to wash regularly with soap and warm water and to avoid greasy cosmetics. In some cases, a course of ultraviolet light treatment may also be recommended. Very dry skin is also a problem that can be inherited; it is caused by reduced sebum production. People with dry skin should avoid washing too much, and avoid harsh soaps. They should use moisturizing creams and emollients, since these seem to be the best remedies for the problem.

Comedones—or blackheads, as they are usually called—are plugs of dry grease and wax that get stuck in the pores of the skin. As a result sebum builds up and can cause the gland to swell into a sebaceous cyst. This can be prevented by squeezing out the blackhead using a special extractor. Blackheads should never be squeezed out with the fingernails, since this could burst any underlying cyst and spread infection. If the blackhead is not removed, the sebum behind it may become infected and produce a boil. When this happens extensively over the skin it is termed "acne" (see Acne and Pimples). The heads of blackheads are black not from dirt but from the oxidation of the outer fatty material that is exposed to the air.

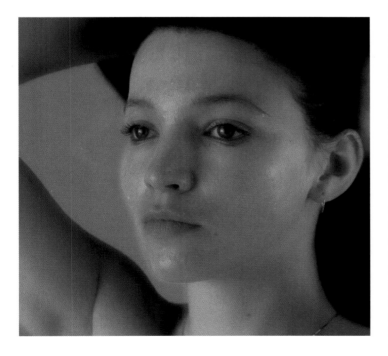

▲ *Sebum provides an effective, natural waterproof layer that prevents skin from becoming too dry.*

See also: **Cosmetics; Hygiene**

Sedatives

Is it true that patients get a sedative injection before surgery?

Yes. This is called premedication; the drug that is usually given is one of the morphine-related drugs. Although these drugs are used principally to relieve pain, they also have a calming effect. The relief of anxiety on the way to the operating room helps to keep patients in a positive state of mind before anesthesia is given and the operation commences.

I find that whenever I am anxious a cup of tea makes me feel better. Is tea a sedative?

Many people find that a cup of tea helps to relieve tension. When you are under greater strain than usual, tea may have a sedating effect. What happens is that you tend to associate a cup of tea with calm and well-being; this association means that the tea is sedative in stressful circumstances. The active substances in tea are in fact stimulant rather than sedative, but the pharmacological (druglike) action is weak, and tea drinking is a harmless habit that many people find very supportive, and a positive boost when they are troubled.

Can you become addicted to sedatives?

Some sedatives are very addictive; barbiturates, for example, are today rarely used as sedatives. Other modern sedatives are not so addictive, but may still be very habit-forming. One way of predicting whether people are likely to make a habit of taking these drugs (in doctors' parlance, become habituated) is to inquire whether they drink a lot of alcohol to help them get over their anxieties. If they do, then habituation is a very real risk; nor should the possibility of alcoholism be discounted.

Only a hundred years ago treatment for severe anxiety might have been a dose of a toxic bromine compound or opium and its derivative, morphine. Nowadays, however, there are many specific, nonaddictive sedatives available.

In a general sense sedatives are drugs that relax and calm people, and so relieve anxiety. Forty years ago, there were only a handful of drugs available that could do this, but now there is a bewildering choice. Sedative drugs are the most commonly prescribed sort of drug in the world, and there is a very real danger that they are overprescribed. Nevertheless, they have been found to be effective and have a definite place in treating people suffering from anxiety and related difficulties such as sleeplessness.

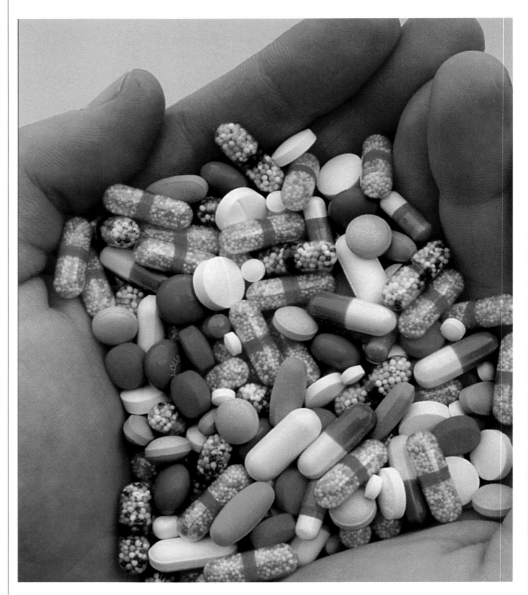

▲ *There is a bewildering array of sedatives available today. Sedative drugs include sleeping drugs, antianxiety drugs, antipsychotic drugs, and some of the antidepressant drugs; worldwide they are the most common form of prescribed drug.*

Sedative drugs work on the brain. The brain is such a complicated structure that it is hardly surprising that sedatives may have other effects beyond simply reducing anxiety. All effective sedatives can also be used as hypnotics (drugs that put people to sleep), provided that a high enough dose is used. Another characteristic of drugs that are truly sedative is that many are very effective in the treatment of epilepsy. For example, diazepam, which is more commonly known as Valium, is used as a standby treatment for people who are having epileptic fits.

Types of sedative

The first important sedatives to be used were opium and alcohol. Opium and its derivatives are rarely prescribed today because of the very high risk of addiction. Alcohol, too, is not often prescribed as a sedative, but it is a tradition in millions of homes that the stresses and strains of work are relieved by a drink at the end of the working day. Although this habit is relatively harmless in people who are not prone to anxiety, it can have damaging effects on anyone who is inclined to worry.

Alcohol can be effective in helping to restore peace of mind, but it is all too easy for someone to depend on alcohol to see him or her through the day. This may quickly lead to physical and psychological addiction (see Alcoholism).

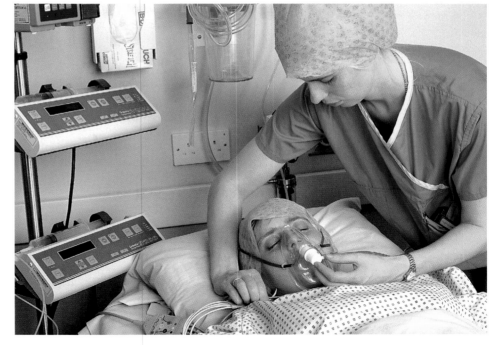

▲ *Patients undergoing surgery are usually given a sedative first to reduce anxiety.*

In the early part of the 20th century, bromides (which have a depressant action on the central nervous system) were widely used as sedatives. However, they had serious side effects; if they were administered over a long period, they caused drowsiness, loss of sensation, and slurred speech. Bromides were replaced as sedatives by barbiturates, which were highly effective in treating anxiety; they also worked as hypnotics and as drugs for epilepsy. They are not prescribed as sedatives or sleeping pills, because they are extremely addictive (see Barbiturates).

The next major group of drugs to be developed were the phenothiazines, which were developed in the early 1950s. The main value of these drugs is as antipsychotics for treating the more serious types of mental disorder such as schizophrenia, but they can also be used to treat anxiety, as can their modern derivatives.

A group of drugs called the benzodiazepines, or tranquilizers, were then developed. The first, chlordiazepoxide (more commonly known as Librium), was made in 1947, but its value in the treatment of anxiety was not recognized and applied until 1964. The benzodiazepines have, in turn, been shown to be as addictive as the barbiturates.

Another major family of drugs that have a sedative action is the antidepressants, which are used mainly to treat depression. It is not uncommon for patients to suffer from a mixture of anxiety and depression, and antidepressants (particularly those known as the tricyclic antidepressants) are

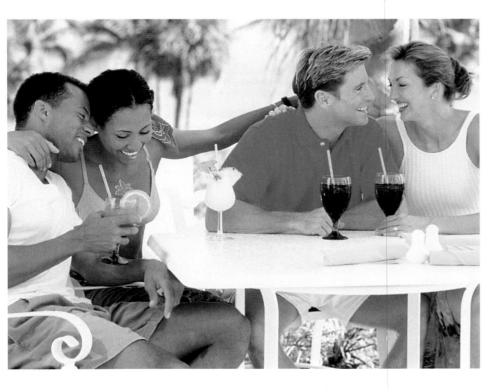

▲ *Alcoholic drinks, in moderation, can act as sedatives and help people to relax. If alcohol is used habitually, there is a risk of alcoholism.*

Questions and Answers

My husband now seems to need at least two alcoholic drinks in the evening to help him unwind. I think it is better to have a drink rather than to take drugs, but my mother says that he will become an alcoholic. Is she right?

Unfortunately she could be right. It is very unwise to become dependent on alcohol; if you are susceptible to this drug, you are at risk of becoming addicted. In your husband's case, drinking at the end of the day's work is probably just a habit. The best way to find out is for him to try to do without a drink for a week or two. If he finds that he still needs alcohol to relax, then it sounds as though he has anxieties that he needs to discuss rather than try to resolve them with alcohol.

My grandmother has begun to wander around the house in the evenings and at bedtime, and she cannot settle down. Would a sedative help?

It sounds as though she is agitated. She may be anxious about something, and it seems that a sedative would be appropriate. However, it is possible that a sedative would only make her worse. This is because it is likely that the basic cause of her trouble is the confusion she finds herself in at the times she starts wandering. If you give her a sedative, which acts by slowing down the functions of the brain, you may end up making her confusion worse rather than better.

My little boy rushes around and gets on my nerves. Can I give him a Valium pill to calm him down?

No. If your child is actually hyperactive, which isn't very likely, then Valium will not be of much help in settling him down. It is wrong, and illegal, to give drugs to people for whom they were not prescribed, and the sort of dose that is suitable for an adult could be extremely dangerous for a young child.

very valuable in treating this type of problem. The sedative action of this group of drugs may be so strong that the high dosages that may be necessary to help patients recover from their depression will also make them feel sleepy. This side effect is not as much of a disadvantage as it sounds, though, since depression is a condition that very often causes sleeplessness in sufferers (see Depression).

Finally, there is a family of drugs called the beta-blockers, whose sedative action is almost a side issue. These are important in treating diseases affecting the heart and the circulation. For example, they are used widely in the treatment of both blood pressure and angina. These drugs help to relieve anxiety, particularly when the symptoms of the condition include sweating and palpitations. They work by blocking the effects of the autonomic nervous system, rather than by acting directly on the brain (see Autonomic Nervous System).

How do sedatives work?

Alcohol and barbiturates work by having a generalized suppressive effect on the action of the nerve cells in the brain. Although we tend to think of alcohol as a drug that exhilarates and liberates, it works by suppressing parts of the brain that act to inhibit various types of behavior. If enough alcohol is drunk it will inhibit brain function until unconsciousness results.

The mechanism by which benzodiazepines or tranquilizers act was not at first understood, though their sedative qualities were easy to demonstrate. In fact, one of the first patients to receive Librium called the investigating doctor within 24 hours of starting on the drug and said that he was without any symptoms for the first time in years.

Careful comparative studies have tended to confirm this action, and animal studies have also provided evidence of their effectiveness. Benzodiazepines have been shown to reduce the aggressive instincts in animals and to provoke them to range wider afield in search of food. This phenomenon is what scientists describe as a reduction in normal anxiety.

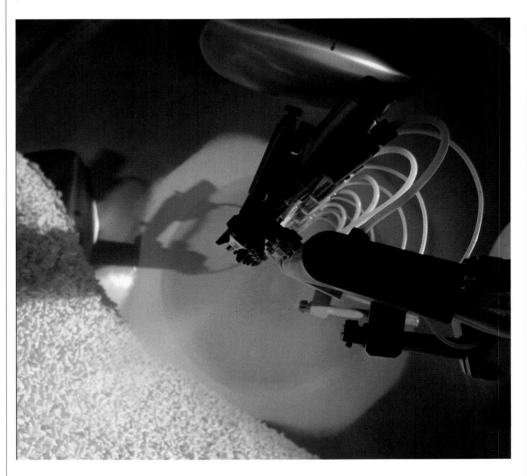

▲ *Many drugs, including sedatives, are coated to make them more palatable and easily identifiable. Here pills are being coated with sugar.*

Are sedatives addictive?

In general, sedatives are addictive. Alcohol, barbiturates, morphine, and heroin are all sedative drugs to some extent, and they are all highly addictive. A physical addiction to benzodiazepines, however, is less common, but they can very easily be habit-forming, so that people who have been taking one of these sedative drugs even for only a week or two may not feel right without them and may soon come to depend on them. Doctors call this psychological addiction (habituation) to distinguish it from a true alteration in the way the body works (which is what happens with morphine or alcohol).

If an anxious person drinks a lot of alcohol to help him or her deal with problems, this is a good indication of the risk of addiction, and many doctors are unwilling to prescribe a benzodiazepine drug to someone who is already dependent on alcohol. Other doctors, however, may feel that benzodiazepines (or tranquilizers) are less of a danger to the body, and that their use is preferable to the risk of allowing the patient to become an alcoholic.

Who needs sedatives?

Anxiety of some sort is an unavoidable part of almost everybody's life. Work, relationships, and sexual anxieties affect all of us at some time and can cause distressing feelings of panic, as well as such physical symptoms as hyperventilation, muscle tension, and gastrointestinal problems.

Doctors have to attempt to determine when anxiety ceases to be

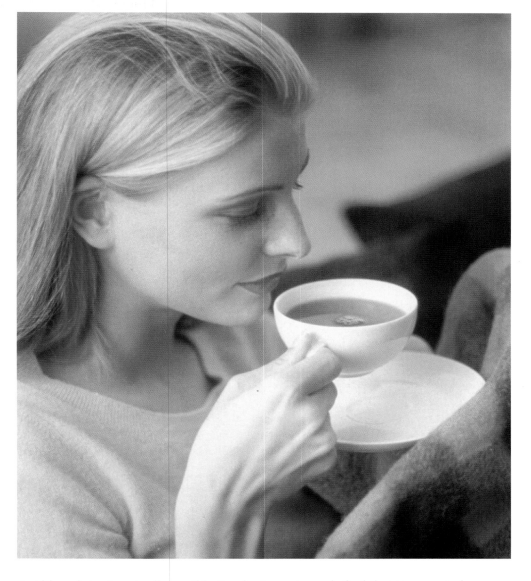

▲ *Although tea is actually a mild stimulant, most people find that it seems to have a sedating effect. They associate it with calm, and find that it helps to relieve simple, everyday tensions.*

normal and becomes a disease. It is not always easy to assess, though the main criteria that a doctor will consider concerns the extent to which anxiety interferes with somebody's life. Even when a doctor decides that a patient does suffer from what is called pathological anxiety, it is by no means definite that drugs will help (see Anxiety). In any case, resolution of the underlying problem, by counseling or by some other kind of psychotherapy, is always preferable to treating a patient with drugs.

Psychoses

However, those suffering from severe psychoses (mental disorders that involve a loss of contact with reality), and in particular schizophrenia and bipolar disorder illnesses (see Bipolar Disorder; Schizophrenia), will generally have to be treated with one of the antipsychotic drugs, such as one of the phenothiazines, thioxanthines, butyrophenones; and other antipsychotics, such as risperidone, olanzapine, quietapine, amisulpride, and zotepine.

Perhaps the main value of sedative drugs is to help someone settle down enough to take stock of a situation and to give him or her a little time to work through the problems, often with the help of some type of counseling.

Which sedative is used?

Usually, the vast majority of people who need either a sedative or a sleeping pill are given one of the benzodiazepine group of drugs. If a doctor thinks that a patient is at risk of becoming habituated to these drugs, he may prefer to prescribe one of the major antipsychotic drugs, such as clozapine.

For patients in the hospital with serious illnesses, or in cases where anxiety arises through pain, morphine or a morphine-based drug may be the best choice of drug.

> *See also:* Counseling; Drug abuse; Insomnia; Morphine; Psychotherapy

Semen

Questions and Answers

My boyfriend argues that the words semen and sperm mean the same thing. I say that the semen contains the sperm so they are different. Which of us is right?

You both are. If you use the word sperm as an abbreviation for spermatozoa—the microscopic swimming cells, one of which can fertilize the female egg and start a pregnancy—then "sperm" is different from "semen." The word "sperm" was used before much was known about spermatozoa and has, for centuries, described the generative substance of males, ejaculated during sexual intercourse; in that context the word means the same as semen.

How do doctors distinguish between "semen" and "sperm"?

When doctors talk about spermatozoa, or about a single spermatozoon, they use the full name or shorten the term to "sperm" or "a sperm." When they talk about seminal fluid, they either use the full phrase or shorten it to semen. They would never call semen "sperm" or confuse it with spermatozoa.

Is semen thick because of the number of sperm in it?

No. Although there are many millions of sperm in an ejaculate; the bulk of the sperm is only a few percent of the total volume.

My brother is worried about wet dreams and thinks there's something wrong with him. He is too embarrassed to talk to anyone but me about it. What can I do?

Explain that sperm are produced all the time. When the pressure gets too high semen is released spontaneously. Most adolescent boys have wet dreams; doctors call them nocturnal emissions.

Semen, or seminal fluid, is the sticky material that forms the ejaculate produced during the male orgasm. It is a complex material that provides a transport medium, a nutritional supply, and an activating factor for the spermatozoa.

There are numerous references to semen in ancient literature, including the Bible, in which it is commonly described as "seed." Semen is a sticky, opalescent fluid that, in addition to the spermatozoa, contains a large number of chemical substances that include sperm nutrients, chemical buffers to protect against vaginal acidity, prostaglandins, substances to increase the motile activity of the sperm, and mucus (see Prostaglandins).

Sources and content

Semen is not fully constituted until just before ejaculation. The spermatozoa are formed in the testicles at the rate of about 30 million each day, and are carried up two tubes, one on each side, called the vasa deferentia. Each tube is called a vas deferens, and is filled with sperm, which form a kind of sludge. Contrary to popular belief, the sperm do not swim up the vas deferens but are pushed up from below by the accumulation of the new sperm that are being produced, and by peristaltic-like contractions of the smooth muscle in the walls of the vasa deferentia. The sperm remain nonmotile until stimulated by chemicals added to the fluid higher up.

The material in the vasa deferentia is not semen. Many constituents must be added before it is complete. The bulk of the fluid in semen comes from the prostate gland and from the adjacent seminal vesicles (see Prostate Gland). The prostate provides most of the additional fluid bulk, but the chemicals that increase sperm motility come from the seminal vesicles. It was once believed

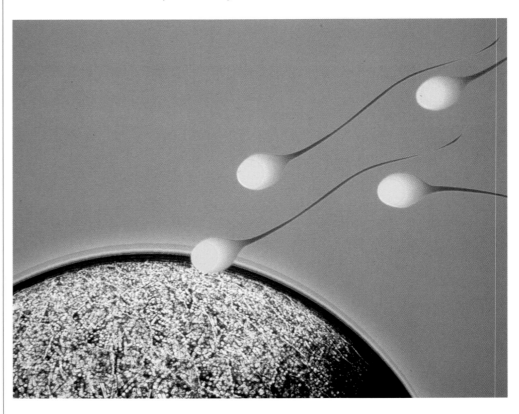

▲ *A graphic illustration of magnified swimming cells or spermatozoa. One of them will fertilize the female ovum (egg).*

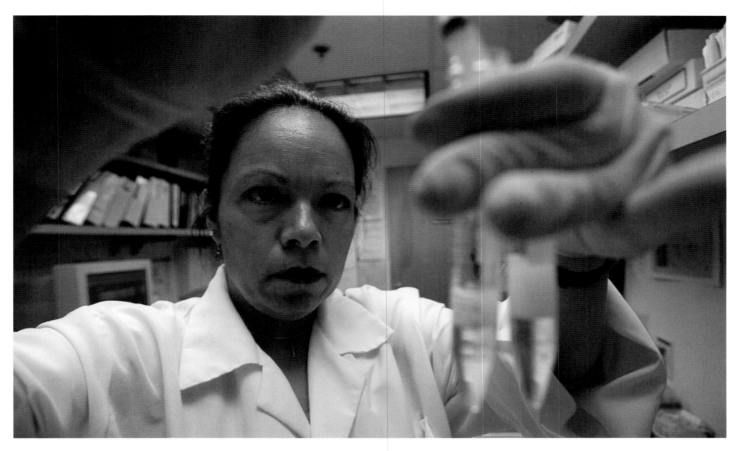

▲ *A lab manager at the Sperm Bank of California collects semen from donors that may later be used in artificial insemination.*

that semen was stored in the seminal vesicles, but this is not the case. The main storage site for sperm awaiting ejaculation are the vasa deferentia. The vesicles are filled with a solution of chemicals waiting to be ejected into the seminal fluid. Substances added to the fluid include choline, phosphocholine, citric acid, and acid phosphatase. The principal nutrient is the sugar fructose.

Formation and ejaculation of semen

The full formation of semen is not complete until shortly before ejaculation occurs; once the semen is fully formed by the addition of secretions from the prostate and seminal vesicles, ejaculation is virtually beyond control. This final stage is brought about by an almost simultaneous contraction of smooth muscle in the testicles, vasa deferentia, prostate gland, and seminal vesicles. This has the effect of mixing all the constituents and forcing the newly formed semen into the rear part of the urethra—the tube running though the prostate gland and penis that, at other times, also carries urine to the exterior.

The urethra has two rings of muscle (sphincters) capable of closing it off. The inner sphincter is immediately below the bladder and above the prostate gland. The outer sphincter lies immediately below the prostate. Expulsion of the semen is completed by a series of rapid, convulsive contractions of the smooth muscle of the urethral wall and the skeletal muscle at the base of the penis and a sudden relaxation of the outer urethral sphincter. The average volume of an ejaculate is about 0.1 fluid ounces (3 ml) and contains up to 300 million spermatozoa. During ejaculation, the sphincter immediately below the bladder is tightened strongly. This prevents urine from being passed during ejaculation and it also prevents semen from passing back and upward into the bladder. Men who have had surgery to remove excess prostate tissue, however, will usually no longer have control over the inner urethral sphincter, so during ejaculation, the semen passes back into the bladder and none is released from the end of the penis. This is called retrograde ejaculation. Although it may result in sterility, it does not affect the sensation of the orgasm.

Sperm quality

Semen looks much the same whether it is fertile or sterile. The difference is mainly in the number and quality of the spermatozoa. This can vary widely from man to man and is influenced by a number of factors. In different men, each 0.03 fluid ounces (1 ml) of semen may contain anything from about 20 million to about 90 million spermatozoa. Any man with a sperm count of less than 20 million per 0.03 fluid ounces (1 ml) is likely to be infertile.

Fertility

Factors other than sperm count can influence fertility; they include lack of adequately vigorous sperm movement, excessive numbers of abnormal forms, and various subtle defects that affect the ability of sperm to fuse with the egg. The investigation of infertility then starts with a detailed study of a sample of semen.

See also: **Conception; Erection and ejaculation; Infertility; Orgasm; Penis and disorders; Sperm; Testes**

Senility

Although the prospect of living to a healthy old age is something to relish, many people are haunted by the specter of senility. As modern medicine discovers more about the process of aging, these fears should recede.

My grandfather, aged 85, has very clear memories about the past, especially his childhood, but cannot remember what happened last week. Is this unusual?

No, not at all. As we get older, it is our short-term memory (our memory for recent events) that fails us first. Older people often tend to dwell on the past: not surprisingly, since it was probably more exciting for them than the present. It seems more real to them than everyday life, to which perhaps they pay less attention than younger people do.

I am 70 and have recently started studying again to get a college degree. I'm enjoying the work, but some of my friends say I'm an old fool. Are they right?

No, they are wrong to undermine your confidence. There is no reason why you should not be successful in your studies; the ability to learn does not decline markedly in later life. You may have to proceed more slowly than you would have done in your earlier years, but that need not detract from your enjoyment in any way. You are wise to keep an active mind and will no doubt retain your mental clarity for many years to come.

My sister and I visit an elderly neighbor who does not seem to have any other visitors. She seems very alert, and she and her house are well cared for. Is she all right?

Your neighbor may prefer to live an independent life. Not all elderly people feel the need for a great deal of company: some disengage or withdraw from society. Since your neighbor seems fit and active, don't worry; just visit her at intervals. She may prefer the company of younger people to that of her peers but is not in a position to seek it out.

Older people are individuals just like everyone else and are entitled to be treated as such, and there is no pattern for old age any more than there is for any other age. Recent research has found that not only individuals, but processes within the individual, age at different rates. Chronological age may well eventually become irrelevant: as more is discovered about the aging process, the individual and his or her doctor can do more to prevent degeneration (see Aging).

Medical attitudes toward old age are changing. Enlightened doctors do not now equate it with illness. It is now understood that confused states of mind in older people, far from being an inescapable feature of advancing years, are often linked to physical illness: once the condition is treated, mental clarity returns. Indeed, confusion can indicate that a physical illness is present.

The needs of the elderly

Older people will suffer more than the general population if the basic necessities of life such as food, heating, shelter, and clothing are not freely available, and most responsible governments throughout the world try to ensure that such needs are provided for their senior citizens.

Satisfying the social needs of the elderly is a more difficult matter. It seems likely that older people would remain more alert, and more active mentally, if they could benefit from company

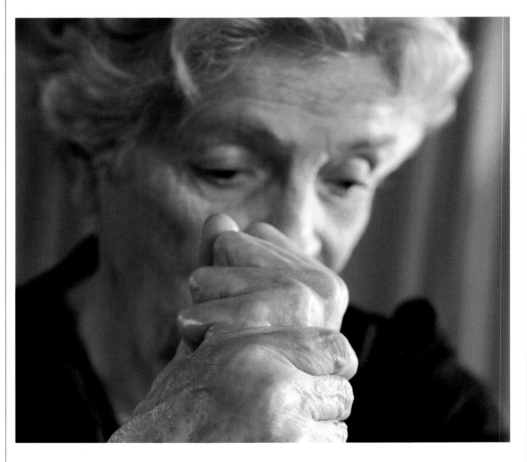

▲ *Alone, incapacitated, and depressed: this is the image of old age we all dread. What we probably fear most is the loss of mental clarity, rather than physical disability.*

in the form of day centers and visits from neighbors and relatives, and take up hobbies. For many, this is undoubtedly the case. However, recent research has shown that there is a tendency in later life to disengage from the community and to withdraw from involvement with the wider world.

Ideally, the image of old age needs to change. In the developed world, which tends to revere youth, age is equated with the feeble, the useless, and decaying. Yet age can be associated with experience, wisdom, and social value. In China, for instance, retirement from paid work was traditionally considered to be a period of active commitment in the form of leading local improvement committees, training young people, and generally putting experience and skills at the service of society. Even in China, however, as traditional society breaks down, the elderly are beginning to suffer the neglect that is so common in Western societies.

The West, which now has a great many citizens between 60 and 80 who are fit and functioning, has to change its approach to old age. Elderly people will have to be given a role and status in society; and while one cannot, of course, quantify the change, a valued place in society should help in turn to bring about improved emotional health in that age group. Many people know of an old person who sinks on retirement into physical or psychiatric illness because he or she cannot cope with a passive role after an active, high-status existence.

How the mind alters
Intellectually and physiologically, people reach a peak in their early twenties, and from then onward there is a decline. However, the decline does not really become obvious until about the age of 70. Intelligence tests indicate that the deterioration in mental powers is most noticeable in those tests that call for logical problem solving. In general, older people appear to become more literal and concrete in their thinking and less able to grasp more abstract concepts. However, research has shown that although many artists and scientists do their major work in their twenties and thirties, they can still make valuable contributions in their fields in their sixties and seventies.

Not all aspects of intelligence decline in the same way. Tests that investigate the use of vocabulary and factual knowledge show little deterioration. Some researchers believe that there should be special intelligence tests for the elderly: they think that older people possess sagacity, which is not the same as intellectual functioning. As one writer phrases it: "Wisdom and intelligence do not necessarily go hand in hand."

Most people notice a general slowing down as they get older. Tests show that this takes place in the central, decision-making processes rather than in muscular capacity or movement: it is our response to signals that slows down rather than our capacity for carrying out movements, although of course there can be some loss of muscular function. Many people complain of failing memory as time goes by. It is generally the short-term memory that is most

▼ *Many older people do not want to enter institutions; they prefer the independence of their own homes. However, homes for the elderly can provide a convivial, healthy, and safe environment for many people, particularly those who are alone or suffering from poor health.*

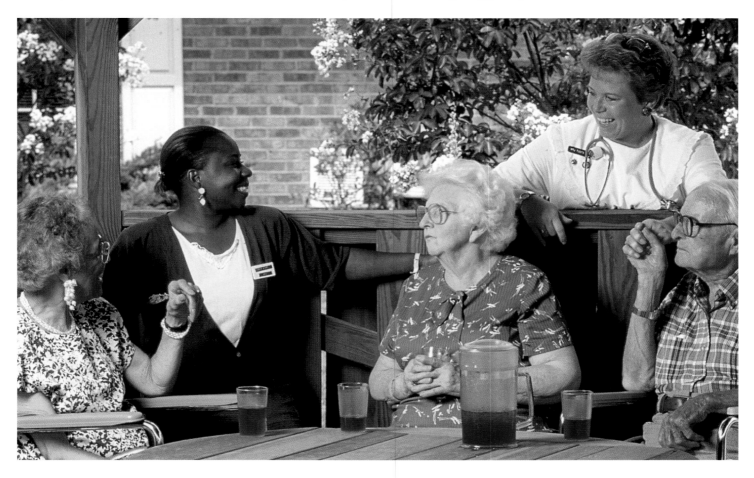

My father-in-law has cancer which is accompanied by a deteriorating mental state. He is being cared for by my mother-in-law, but he is difficult to nurse. My husband thinks he should be in the hospital, but his mother says this is heartless. What do you think?

I think it would probably be better for your father-in-law to be in the hospital. Not only will it provide more facilities for nursing, but it will prevent your mother-in-law's own health from suffering if she continues to keep him at home. I'm sure your father-in-law would not wish to be a burden on his wife or to be the cause of a decline in her health. If your mother-in-law insists on nursing him, her doctor may arrange for nursing help and support. You and the other younger relatives could also help her out.

My elderly mother went into the hospital with a heart condition. After surgery, she seemed disoriented. What went wrong?

Nothing necessarily went wrong. It is recognized today that physical conditions, such as heart disease, and also hospital treatment, such as surgery and anesthesia, can give rise to temporary confusion, particularly in elderly patients. As your mother recovers from her heart condition and from the operation you will probably find that she will regain her mental clarity.

I am only 50, but I find I am beginning to forget names of people and places. Is this the first step toward senility?

Many people worry when their memory fails them, but it is important to remember that our long-term memory and our ability to learn may remain intact well into our eighties, if not longer.

If you are bothered by your forgetfulness, get into the habit of taking notes, and learn about or invent your own ways of reminding yourself of things you want to remember.

affected. Long-term memory seldom presents problems, although there may be times when older people have difficulty in recalling facts when they need to remember them.

Despite what many people think, the ability to learn does not decline radically with age. Research shows that older people show the least decline in this ability when they are faced with learning-associated facts; they are disadvantaged when the facts are unrelated or when the material is mainly theoretical. On the positive side, elderly people have a wealth of experience. This is an attribute that can enrich both the individual's personal life and that of society.

Impairment of faculties

It has to be accepted that some loss of faculties is common in old age, and it is wise to be aware of what these may be so that remedial action can be taken. Much distress and discomfort could be avoided if people took medical advice promptly on finding that their eyesight or hearing, for example, was slightly impaired, rather than waiting until the condition was serious.

One of the characteristic changes in the eye is that viewing distance gradually lengthens until, at the age of 50 or so, many people need to wear glasses to correct this farsightedness. Hearing loss is usually gradual and affects higher tones more than lower ones. With age the voice becomes more highly pitched and speech slower. The sense of taste changes, with a decrease in sensitivity to salt and sugar; the sense of smell may atrophy; and tolerance of pain may decrease. It must be stressed, however, that not all the faculties decline together. There are marked individual differences; some people retain most or even all their faculties into their eighties and even their nineties.

Psychiatric disorders

Mental disorders in older people are often classified into four kinds: delirious and confusional states, depression, paraphrenia, and organic psychoses. Delirious and confusional states in an elderly patient can be a sign of acute physical illness. Confusion is characterized by an

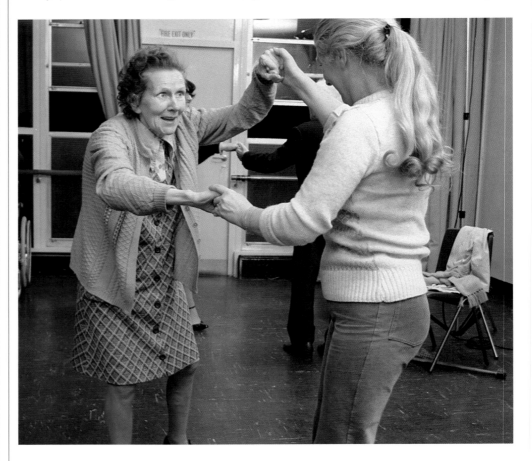

▲ *For elderly people, dancing can be fun. It also provides much needed exercise for someone who is probably sedentary for most of the time.*

► *While some elderly people suffer physical or psychiatric impairment, and may consequently require care either in the home or within an institution, many older people enjoy practicing many different handicrafts and hobbies. Talking and reminiscing with congenial and sympathetic people is also important to an elderly person.*

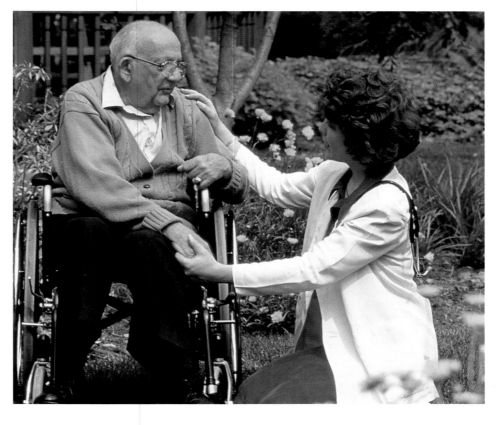

individual's becoming muddled and disoriented; if someone is suffering from delirium, there may be hallucinations as well. These states tend to be temporary. The physical causes of the disorder can often be strokes or heart disease, but minor infections like cystitis; more severe illnesses such as bronchitis, pneumonia, or anemia; or drugs or anesthesia may exacerbate the problem. Treatment for confusional states involves treatment of the underlying illness.

Among the many affective psychoses, depression is the most common and may take the form of endogenous depression (a biochemical disorder) or depression caused by such factors as loneliness, bereavement, or retirement. Older people can be treated for depression in exactly the same way as younger people, and many respond very well (see Depression).

Late paraphrenia is a psychosis similar to schizophrenia in which the older person develops paranoid delusions while otherwise remaining mentally alert and physically healthy. Often the individual can live satisfactorily with his or her fantasies and continue to live a useful life within the community.

Organic psychoses fall into two types: senile psychosis (senile dementia) and arteriosclerotic psychosis. Both involve a slow breakdown of personality, which ends in dementia; both are the result of degenerative processes at work in the brain (see Alzheimer's Disease).

Senile psychosis is characterized by a gradual unremitting deterioration; whereas the patient with arteriosclerotic psychosis may have remissions of seemingly complete mental clarity. There is no treatment at present for these psychoses, but attention to routine, personal hygiene, mental stimulus in the form of company, and hobbies can all help the individual in the early stages.

Approaches to old age

Everyone can take a positive attitude to advancing age, both his or her own age and that of other people. How people are when they are old depends to a great extent on how they were when they were younger. It is never too early to develop good habits of diet and regular exercise which can be continued into later life. Obesity and inactivity are the enemies of good health in old age. Even when people are in their forties and fifties, they can prepare for leisure in retirement by cultivating hobbies and interests. Volunteer work is an activity that can be carried out at almost any age. Many people find that they discover what life is about only after they retire.

It can be helpful for people to keep reminding themselves that being old is partly a psychological matter. If older people aim to be active, stay interested in their surroundings, and are of use to the community, their biological age is irrelevant.

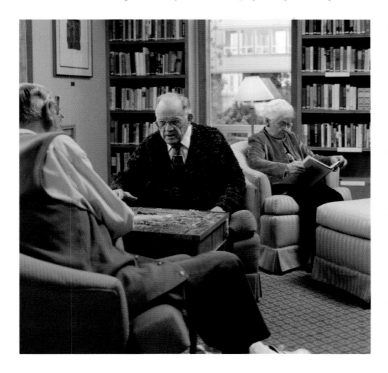

▲ *Retirement homes aim to keep elderly people stimulated by activities that keep their minds active.*

See also: **Dementia**

Sensitization

Sensitization is the process by which we build up immunity to disease and develop allergies. Allergy sufferers can benefit by exploiting this process through an organized program of desensitization.

Sensitization is the process by which the body becomes sensitive to a foreign substance. It is a vital part of our immune system, ensuring that once we have a disease, such as chicken pox, we build up a defense against it and can fight off future attacks (see Immune System). However, "sensitization" is a term more commonly used to describe the emergence of an allergy.

Occasionally, the immune system goes wrong and someone develops a sensitivity to a substance that does not normally cause any harm. The allergic reaction, as in hay fever, food allergies, and asthma, can be most unpleasant (see Allergies).

There are a number of methods for dealing with an allergy. Avoiding the substance and taking antihistamine and steroid drugs are methods commonly used, but both have disadvantages. Desensitization offers another option that can sometimes give more effective relief.

Desensitization

Desensitization is a method sometimes used to reduce or eliminate a person's sensitivity to a given substance. It does not work for everyone but it is worth trying because it offers considerable advantages over the more traditional methods. It is actually very similar to the process of sensitization, which is how the allergy comes about in the first place, but has the opposite effect and involves the immune system in a way that is not clearly understood.

Sensitization

Sensitization occurs when a person is exposed repeatedly to varying strengths of allergen (a substance that causes an allergic reaction) over a period of time. The fluctuation of the strength of the allergen and the irregularity of exposure to it appear to have some bearing on the emergence of the allergy. In striking contrast, a desensitization program works because it is

Questions and Answers

I recently reacted to penicillin and have been told I am sensitized to it. How could this be, since I have never had penicillin?

We do not know why one person is sensitive to a substance and another is not. In the case of penicillin, you may have been given it under an unfamiliar drug name. Farmers used to include penicillin in cattle feed to improve the milk yield, and the penicillin was then in the milk, so you could have been sensitized through drinking cows' milk.

I get hay fever every year and nothing relieves it. Could desensitization give me relief?

Desensitization for hay fever can be successful. The underlying mechanism of the treatment is not fully understood, but the full course of injections can give at least one season free of hay fever. It does not work for everyone; others may have a long-lasting or even a permanent cure.

Desensitization must be done under carefully controlled conditions, with resuscitation facilities near at hand, because of the danger of fatal reactions.

I found that I am sensitive to many substances. Can I be desensitized against all of them?

Yes, and all at once. Once the doctor knows what you are sensitive to and decides on your program of desensitization, he or she sends the details to a special laboratory. It makes up a solution containing dilute traces of all the substances to which you are allergic. This solution is injected in graduated steps and may reduce or eliminate all your sensitivities. If you react to any of the substances, the course will be stopped, the allergen responsible for the reaction traced, and the cocktail changed accordingly.

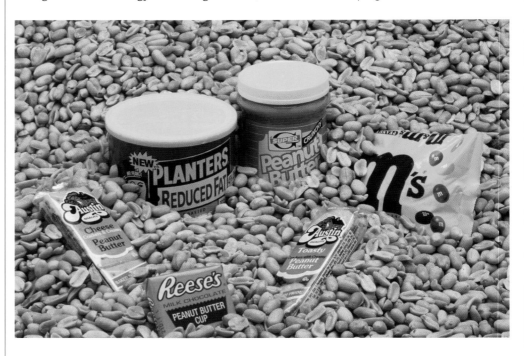

▲ *Peanuts are one of the most allergenic foods. For someone sensitive, it is a lifelong allergy and even trace amounts can be fatal.*

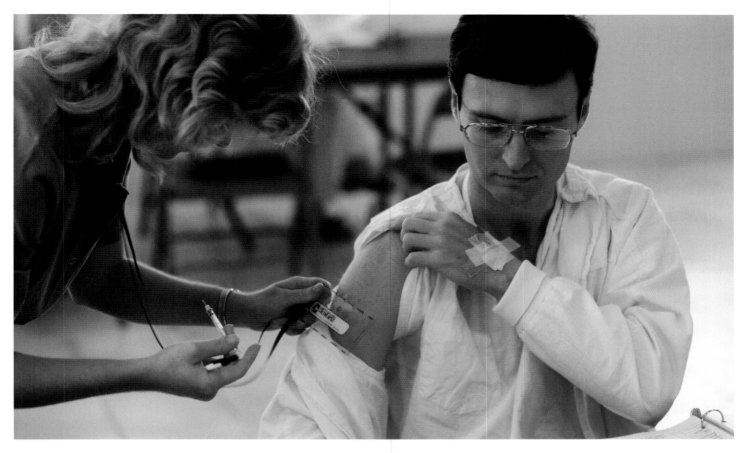

▲ *Allergy testing is carried out in sterile conditions in a hospital cleanroom.*

carefully planned. Gradually increasing doses of the substance to which the body is allergic are injected at regular intervals. This has the effect of building up a tolerance to the substance. However, if the carefully planned program is broken at any stage, or if too strong a dose is given too soon, the body may react strongly, and develop an allergic reaction similar to the original problem.

Identifying allergens

First the underlying cause of the allergic reaction is diagnosed. This is established through a number of different tests. The prick test is usually used for asthma and various types of hay-fever allergies. A doctor pricks the arm with a needle and then introduces a number of different allergens. Up to 40 of these pinpricks may be made in one session. A red welt shows up if a person is allergic to any of the allergens. In the patch test, which is often used for skin-contact sensitivities, weak solutions of the suspected allergens are left on the arm and covered. After 48 hours the area is inspected for reaction. The severity of the reaction indicates the person's degree of sensitivity to the allergen. This is important because the doctor can then establish the first dose in the desensitization program.

Treatment

If a person is allergic to a number of substances, then all of these can be treated at the same time in the same way. A special solution is prepared containing traces of all the substances to which the person is allergic. The first dose is critical; the solution must be as strong as

possible without producing a reaction. The patient is injected and returns the following week for a further injection. If there is a reaction at this or any time, or if the course of treatment is broken, then the course must be restarted. This first injection is followed by a further series: each dose is a slightly stronger solution than the previous one until, at the completion of the course, the patient is desensitized and shows no reaction to the allergen. In effect, the allergy has disappeared.

Desensitization injections can never be assumed to be entirely safe. Current medical practice requires that any doctor performing desensitization must be equipped to carry out emergency resuscitation including the passage of a tracheal tube for emergency ventilation. He or she must also have appropriate drugs available for injection, including epinephrine and high-dosage steroids.

Practical uses

The most common use of this method is in desensitizing sufferers of hay fever or asthma caused by pollen or the dust mite (see Asthma). In the case of hay fever the course of injections should be taken before the pollen season starts; the treatment is usually less reliable if the injections are given during the season. It may not work for everybody, but it offers 70 percent of sufferers protection through the season. It is not a guaranteed or a permanent cure, so the treatment may have to be repeated the following year, but this varies from one person to another. Research on food allergies continues. In the future it may be possible to treat them using techniques similar to those described above.

See also: **Hay fever; Shock**

Sepsis

Questions and Answers

Who is at risk from sepsis?

Anyone is potentially at risk of severe sepsis after catching an infection, but it is the very young, the very old, hospital patients, and those who already have medical conditions who are most at risk. Some common factors that increase the chance of triggering severe sepsis are an underactive immune system, for example from chemotherapy or immunosuppressor medicines used after organ transplants; recent surgery; genetics; and using an IV drip, a catheter, or another procedure that invades the body.

Why does severe sepsis happen?

When a person becomes infected, the body's immune system acts to fight the invading bacteria or other infective agents. The body usually regulates its response to infection with chemicals called immune modulators. Sometimes the infection and other toxins cause the production of too many modulators, which inflame the body's blood vessels, causing the release of yet more immune modulators. The body goes into severe sepsis as the immune reaction spirals out of control, causing inflammation and clotting throughout the body's organs and blood system. This inflammation and clotting can lead to failure of the vital organs, from which the patient will die unless treated.

Where in the body does sepsis usually occur?

An infection in any part of the body can cause severe sepsis but the most common sources are: the lungs, the gut or bowels; the skin through wounds or invasive devices like IV drips; the urinary tract from catheters, with possible spread to the bladder or kidneys; and the brain or spinal cord.

The body's response to infection from invading bacteria, viruses, or other infective agents is called sepsis. In severe sepsis this response goes out of control, causing inflammation and damage throughout the body's organs and blood system that can kill the patient.

Sepsis can be a very severe and life-threatening illness. It can cause organ failure or even a catastrophic drop in blood circulation. According to the National Institutes of Health about one in 50 hospital admissions is from sepsis, and sepsis affects more than 750,000 Americans a year. Further, in its most severe cases the mortality rate can be as high as 50 percent. Sepsis is also called systematic immune response syndrome (SIRS).

Different types of sepsis

There are several different types of sepsis that are classified according to their severity and effect. A patient can have sepsis that progresses from one type to another as the disease worsens—for example, when the sepsis starts, it may be uncomplicated; it may progress to severe and then to septic shock.

Uncomplicated sepsis: This is caused by flu, gastroenteritis, or other common infections. It affects millions of people every year and is usually not serious.

Severe sepsis: If the sepsis is complicated by problems in the vital organs it is said to become severe. The condition is then life-threatening, with a mortality rate of around 30 percent.

Septicemia: When an infection of the blood, called blood poisoning, becomes out of control the sepsis leads to septicemia. If allowed to worsen it can cause septic shock.

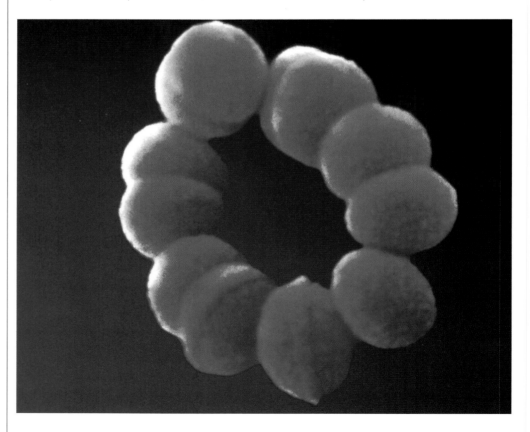

▲ *Streptococcus bacteria, which are responsible for causing many diseases, are shown here as a colorized electron micrograph that is magnified 7,000 times.*

Septic shock: This is a serious condition that happens when an infection leads to a dramatic drop in blood flow and potential organ damage or failure. Its mortality rate is around 50 percent.

Sources of infection

Any infection, anywhere in the body can lead to severe sepsis. If a patient has pneumonia, the lungs can be the source of the infection, and in cases of appendicitis or bowel and gallbladder infections, sepsis can be triggered. Other common sources are wounds in the skin or invasive devices such as intravenous lines or cannulas; catheters in the urinary tract, through which infection can spread to the bladder or kidneys; and infections of the brain or spinal cord, such as meningitis or encephalitis. In about one in five patients suffering from severe sepsis, the source of the infection is never discovered.

Symptoms and signs

Sepsis has several symptoms that are caused by the body's response to an infection; they include fever or low body temperature (hypothermia); hyperventilation, or an increased breathing rate; rapid heartbeat (tachycardia); decreased urine output; chills; shaking; warm skin; skin rash; confusion or delirium; diarrhea; and nausea or vomiting. Patients who go into septic shock can also show further symptoms, such as shortness of breath, feeling light-headed, heart palpitations, and cool, pale hands and feet.

Doctors can employ several tests to verify whether a patient has severe sepsis, such as measuring to see if the white blood cell count is too high or too low; examining a blood culture for bacteria; and testing for abnormal kidney or liver function. Other tests for septic shock include: measuring blood pressure to see if it is low; doing a chest X ray to reveal pneumonia or pulmonary edema; and carrying out blood tests to show organ dysfunction or failure.

Treatment and care

Patients with severe sepsis or septic shock are seriously ill and may require treatment in an intensive care unit. The most important part of the treatment is to identify and act against the underlying source of infection. At the same time, doctors treat the symptoms and complications from the sepsis itself.

Initially, doctors give a selection of antibiotics to treat a wide range of possible infections. They then try to find both the source and the infection type. If the source is the result of human action, such as a bullet or an infected surgical tube, then it must be removed; if it is an abscess it can be surgically drained. Finally, a more specific antibiotic is used once the type of infection is known, as this helps to lessen the chance of creating drug-resistant bacteria (see Bacteria).

All patients suffering from septic shock need treatment in an intensive care unit, but only some with severe sepsis require such care. To treat the symptoms of sepsis requires particular measures for each problem. An IV drip replaces fluids or supplies nutrients. Vasopressor drugs raise blood pressure. Further, if vital organs are failing, mechanical organ support is needed, such as a dialysis machine for the kidneys or a mechanical ventilator for the lungs.

The future

In recent decades, the number of cases of severe sepsis has quadrupled in the United States. New research is aimed at finding innovative methods of treating or preventing sepsis to combat this alarming rise (see Infection and Infectious Diseases).

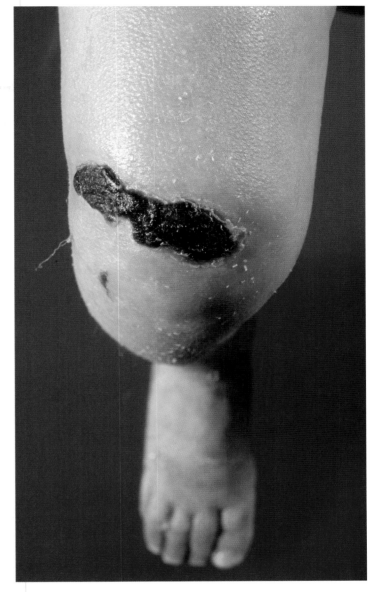

▲ *This skin ulcer on the knee lasted six weeks and then developed severe sepsis that involved the iliac arteries and femoral veins.*

One new drug for treating sepsis is a bioengineered version of activated protein C, a protein that regulates blood clotting and controls inflammation. Many of the symptoms of severe sepsis and septic shock are caused when the body's clotting and inflammation mechanisms spiral out of control, and this drug should help stop such damaging clots from forming in the vital organs. Studies show that it reduces the mortality rate of patients with very severe sepsis from 30 percent to 25 percent. Although modest as a percentage, this is a significant reduction in the large number of patients with sepsis. Another line of research is to develop a sepsis vaccine to prevent the overreaction of the body's immune system (see Immune System). Current animal trials are promising, but it could be a decade before such vaccines are used in hospitals.

> **See also: Intensive care unit**

Sex

Questions and Answers

How many times a week should a couple make love?

It really is a question of what the partners prefer. Some like to have sex every day, others every few weeks, others somewhere in between. If both you and your partner are happy with your own frequency of lovemaking, then don't worry. But if one of you feels unhappy about it, and wants to make love more often (or less often), it is worthwhile having a frank discussion in which you can get to understand the other's needs a little better.

Is it true that there are certain lovemaking positions in which a woman is more likely to conceive?

Each time a man ejaculates he releases millions of sperm, all with the same objective: to swim energetically toward an egg they can fertilize. The lovemaking position is unlikely to make much difference, as long as the man ejaculates well inside the vagina.

Some friends talked about multiple orgasms. What are they?

A multiple orgasm is a sequence of mini-orgasms which may occur at the end of a woman's plateau phase, and ends in a powerful climax. Not every woman has multiple orgasms, but they are not necessary for sexual pleasure.

My boyfriend says I don't love him because I don't want to make love. I'm only 16, and feel I'm too young for a sexual relationship. Should I sleep with him or not?

If you don't feel ready for a sexual relationship, don't start one. It doesn't mean that you love your boyfriend any less. He ought to be able to understand that and to see that putting pressure on you will only make you miserable.

From the first yearnings of adolescence, sex plays a major role in our lives; indeed, it is one of our strongest drives. However, for some, what should be a rich source of pleasure can also cause great unhappiness.

Sex is a fundamental driving force of human life, but the complex relationships between the biological need to reproduce, cultural influences, love, affection, and the sex drive are still not fully understood. Much of what we know about human sexuality has been researched and written about during the 20th century, and there is still great controversy about many aspects.

As our society has developed, much of what was once considered taboo is now part of normal sexual behavior and can be discussed freely. In the past a common premise was that women

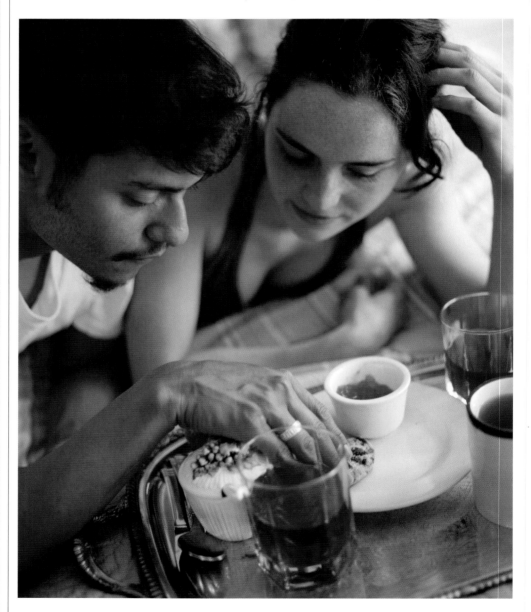

▲ *Interest in the opposite sex usually starts at adolescence or even earlier. Sexual attraction is controlled by factors such as physical appearance and social influences.*

were interested in sex only for the sake of fulfilling a maternal instinct or pleasing their partners. It has now become clear that women have as powerful a need for sexual satisfaction and fulfilment as men. Men used to be seen as less emotional and sensitive, wanting sex only to gratify some basic animal urge, but we now know that emotional expression in sexual activity is equally important to men and women.

Sexual awareness

Our first conscious expression of interest in sex may come with the question "Where do babies come from"? but, in fact, we are sexual animals from birth. We enjoy and are aware of a variety of physical sensations, many of which represent the warmth and comfort of closeness with another person. We get sensual pleasure from our bodies long before we are aware of ourselves as sexual beings or what sexual pleasure means in society.

Sexual interest in other people may not arise until adolescence begins, although it may happen considerably earlier. Surveys now suggest that the majority of young people are sexually experienced by the time they have reached the age of 18.

Sexual attraction

What attracts people sexually to each other? The answer to this question can be split to cover three broad areas: physical factors, psychological factors, and social influences. On a physiological level, much depends on what a prospective sexual partner looks like, not simply in the sense of physical appearance, but more in terms of whether he or she looks interested or available. It has been suggested that if the pupils of the eyes of someone who is being looked at dilate as he or she is spoken to, this signifies attraction, or at least interest.

Smell also plays a part, though it may be heavily disguised or register only at an unconscious level. Like all animals, humans produce subtle scents called pheromones, which may be a powerful influence on sexual attraction.

On the psychological level, it is true to say that everybody judges potential sexual partners on a wide range of factors, including likeness or dissimilarity to his or her mother or father. Social influences are very important. Everyone is constantly assaulted with images of how the ideal sex partner ought to look, act, and live; and there is little doubt that these factors can greatly influence

▼ *Pierce Brosnan and Halle Berry star in the James Bond movie* Die Another Day. *Our views and expectations of sexuality are formed by countless factors, such as an uninhibited approach to nudity during childhood, the physical pleasures of dancing, and media representations of sex and romance.*

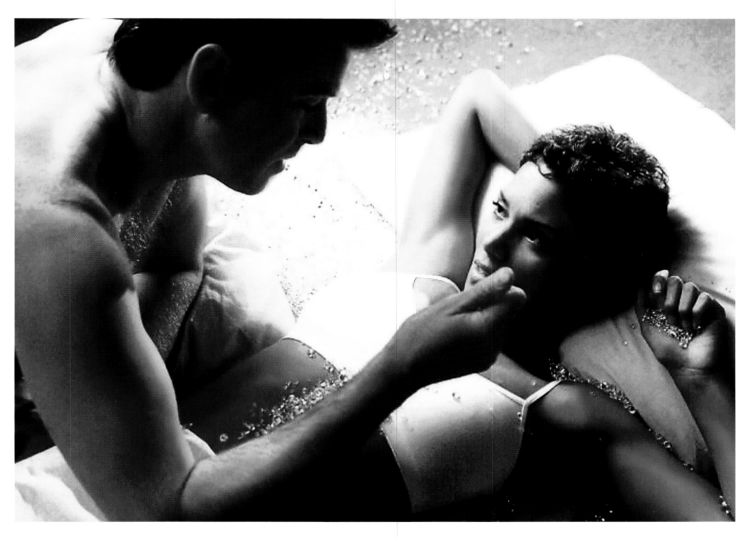

Questions and Answers

My daughter is 14 and has started going out with boys. My husband and I have given her permission to do this, but we are still worried about her. Is 14 too young?

That depends on how physically and psychologically mature your daughter is and what kind of relationships she is involved in. It is very important to keep communication open with your daughter so that she feels able to confide in you and you feel able to tell her what you think about her relationships. You cannot stop your daughter from growing up and it is completely natural for her to have close relationships outside the family.

I am no longer lubricated enough before intercourse, and this is interfering with my enjoyment. Is there something physically wrong with me? This started a few months ago, and I am beginning to get quite tense and anxious.

It is very unlikely that there is anything physically wrong with you, but it is worth seeing your doctor to check that all is well. It may be that you and your partner are hurrying sex and rushing into intercourse before you really want to. So relax and try to set the pace yourself, and don't have intercourse until you feel that you are ready for it. If you do not do this, and merely continue at the same pace, you will only make yourself even more tense. Once you are able to overcome this, then almost certainly you will be able to solve your problem.

I have been told by several people that I ought to be circumcised for medical reasons, and that it could improve my sexual performance. Is there any truth in this?

If you believe that it will help, then it actually may help. However, although a man who has been circumcised may have slightly less sensation in the glans (head) of his penis, there is no indication that he is a better or worse lover as a result.

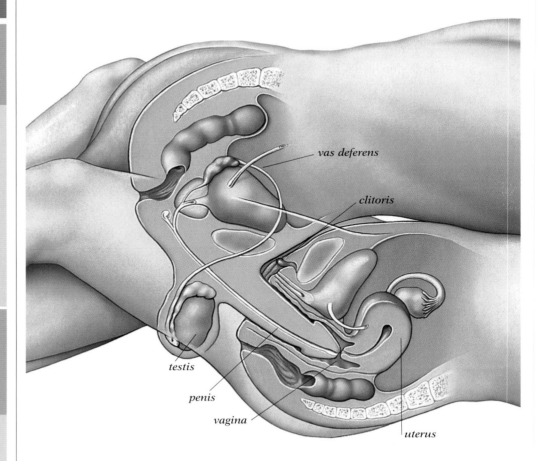

vas deferens

clitoris

testis

penis

vagina

uterus

▲ *Intercourse can take place only when the man has achieved an erection. If the woman is ready and sufficiently lubricated, the penis is guided into her vagina. Through rhythmic movements, excitement increases until orgasm is eventually reached.*

preference. These aspects of sexuality have a great influence throughout adult life and are central to a fulfilling and satisfying sex life.

The female orgasmic cycle

Orgasm is a simple reflex response to sexual stimulation and can occur as the result of a variety of sexual stimuli. The physical cycle of arousal, however, is always exactly the same. The intensity of the experience may vary from woman to woman, and from time to time, and depend on the source of stimulation.

The American sexologists Masters and Johnson identified four phases of the orgasmic cycle: excitement, plateau, orgasm, and resolution.

The excitement phase is brought about by sexual thoughts, by emotional closeness, and by physical attraction. The body immediately reacts to these stimuli with an increase in general sensitivity and response to caresses. The sexual organs become filled with blood, so that they swell both internally and externally.

The vagina expands in length and width, and the vulva swells a little (see Vagina). Both the clitoris and the labia minora (inner lips of the vulva) fill with blood and may become darker in color. The vagina begins to lubricate itself in readiness for sexual contact.

The plateau phase follows immediately. The sexual organs become extremely sensitive, responding to the caresses of lovemaking (see Intercourse). The vagina expands to become about 2 inches (5 cm) longer than it is in the nonaroused state. It is at this point that intercourse may be taking place, and sensation for the man and woman is increased by the narrowing of the outer third of the vagina, making it grip the penis more easily. Lubrication of the vagina

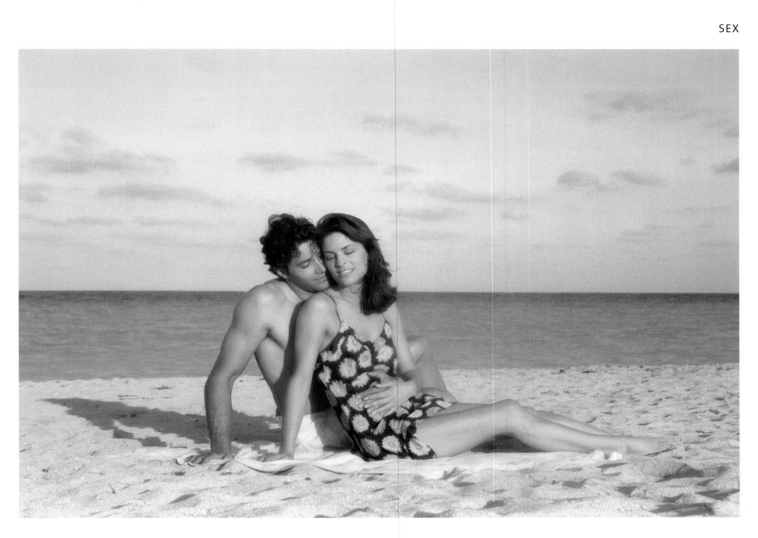

▲ *Keeping fit and having a healthy relationship is one way to help maintain libido and a satisfying sex life.*

continues, and all the muscles around the sexual organs become tense in a pleasurable way. The breasts may swell and the nipples become erect, especially if they are touched. Breathing is deep, and there may be a light rash over the upper parts of the body.

The clitoris, which is the most sensitive of the female sexual organs and is where all orgasms begin, is now fully erect. Just before orgasm it pulls itself back inside the clitoral hood.

Orgasm may now occur. There will be a rush of extremely pleasurable sensations beginning at the clitoris and moving outward into the whole body. The muscles that surround the vulva, vagina, and anus now enter into a series of spontaneous rhythmic contractions. The resolution phase then begins immediately after orgasm. In this phase the sexual organs return to a nonaroused state. The volume of blood that engorged the sexual organs slowly drains away into the rest of the body. Sexual interest may be aroused again almost immediately, and the orgasmic cycle will recommence.

The male orgasmic cycle

The male orgasmic cycle goes through exactly the same sequence: excitement, plateau, orgasm, and resolution. It is equally complex.

The excitement phase begins as a response to a sexual thought or feeling, or to physical stimulation. The penis responds almost immediately, becoming erect (see Penis and Disorders). Blood fills the spaces (corpora cavernosa) within the flaccid (soft) penis, so that it can enlarge to 6 inches (15 cm) or more in length when erect. Breathing deepens, the pulse rate increases, and the body is more sensitive.

The plateau phase follows. The penis is now fully erect, it may have darkened in color, and a drop of liquid may appear at the entrance to the urethra. This is not seminal fluid, but it may contain a few sperm. The testicles increase in size by as much as 50 percent, rising up toward the body. The genital area increases in sensitivity as orgasm is approached.

Orgasm is made up of two stages, but these are linked in such a way that it is impossible to have the first without its being followed immediately by the second. First, sperm are pushed up the vas deferens (seminal duct) to the level of the seminal vesicles. These vesicles produce a fluid, which is mixed with the sperm, and is then ready for ejaculation. About four seconds later, the fluid is pushed into and along the urethra, as a result of a series of contractions made by the prostate gland and the urethral muscles. The semen is then ejaculated out of the urethra, causing a spasm of pleasure.

The resolution phase sees the penis returning to a nonaroused state and losing the erection. The physical tension that has accompanied arousal now disappears, and the man may feel very relaxed.

Physical problems for women

Many women experience sexual problems, particularly with orgasm. A woman may be unable to move from the plateau phase into

How common are sexual problems?

No large-scale survey has ever been done. However, some published results indicate that 40 percent of men and 60 percent of women have suffered some form of difficulty with intercourse, and that 50 percent of men and 77 percent of women have had some form of sexual problem.

Are women ever really frigid, or are they just not turned on by their partners?

A small proportion of women find sexual arousal impossible under any circumstance. Most women who wonder if they are frigid can become aroused with the right man or while masturbating: their difficulty is psychological, not physical. Because of this, the word "frigid" is seldom used medically.

Is there something wrong with men who habitually go to prostitutes?

Apart from any moral issues, not necessarily. Some go because they have difficulty in acquiring a steady girlfriend, others because they have some special ritual or fantasy which they want to play out but which is distasteful to their regular partner.

In sex manuals and some magazines, it is said that the size of the man's penis does not matter. Is this really true?

Yes. Many men become obsessed with the size of their penis to the detriment of their sex lives. An apparently small, flaccid penis often becomes proportionally much larger on erection so that most erect penises are roughly similar in size. Also, the source of most sexual sensations in women is the clitoris and, to a lesser extent, the first third of the vagina, so having a particularly long penis inside will not produce any extra sensation for a woman; it may even cause a woman discomfort.

orgasm, which can be very frustrating. She may be able to reach a climax easily from masturbation, but does not do so as a result of intercourse. This is now thought to be perfectly normal, and may in fact apply to a sizable proportion (a third or more) of all women. Problems with orgasm when a woman is with a partner can sometimes be due to the fact that the woman or her partner does not know how best she can be sexually stimulated to the point of climax; a straightforward sex manual can usually help the couple with this problem. There are, however, a number of physical factors that can lead to sexual problems, and these should be considered before partners go on to seek psychological help with any sexual difficulty.

Libido

Libido is the interest in or need for sex, so it is obviously a prerequisite of enjoyable sexual activity. There are a number of simple problems that can lead to a decrease in libido, but these are often easily rectified (see Libido). Many women report that they have little interest in sex immediately after the birth of a child. This may be a result of the change in hormone levels during and after pregnancy, but it may also be caused simply by physical tiredness. The Pill can

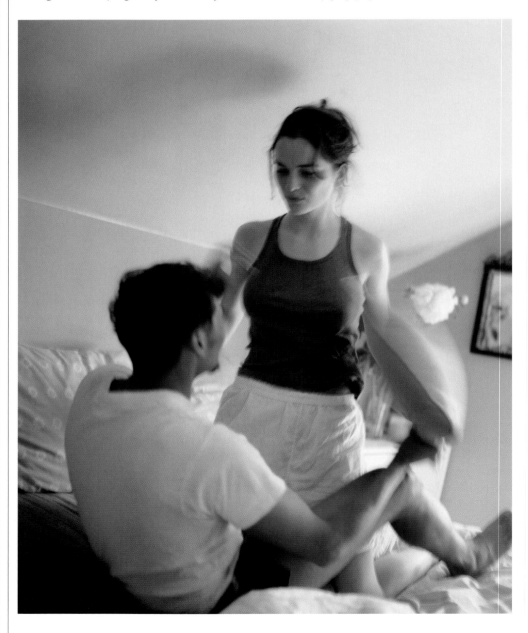

▲ *The excitement of undressing and sexual foreplay before intercourse can add to the arousal of both the man and the woman during the process of lovemaking.*

also reduce libido. This is a relatively uncommon effect and may be easily solved by a change of Pill or by trying a different kind of contraceptive. Once again it is the change in hormone levels that is thought to be responsible for a lessening of libido.

The menstrual cycle can be accompanied by changes in the level of sexual interest. This should not present a problem once the woman and her partner have understood and accepted these cyclical changes. A small minority of women, however, will experience loss of libido as a result of a hormone deficiency or imbalance that is independent of the menstrual cycle, and this needs treatment.

Physical difficulties with arousal and intercourse can also occur as a result of pregnancy and childbirth. The vagina may be very tender after giving birth, and intercourse should not be attempted until all stitches have healed completely. Once vaginal soreness has disappeared (this may take three weeks or more), intercourse can take place as usual.

Painful intercourse needs medical investigation and treatment, because it may indicate gynecological problems, such as cysts on the ovaries or an infection inside the uterus.

Physical problems for men

Although the majority of male sexual problems are psychologically based, there are a number of physical conditions that can affect a man's sex life. It is important for a man to contact his doctor as soon as possible before anxiety over sexual performance begins to complicate matters and create tension.

Genital abnormalities are extremely rare, but when they do occur they can be very upsetting. A tight foreskin can make intercourse painful; an undescended testicle, though it will not affect intercourse, may cause embarrassment. Both of these conditions can be corrected by surgery. Any rash or soreness on the penis will make intercourse uncomfortable and should be treated immediately, either by a doctor or at a special treatment clinic.

MALE AND FEMALE ORGASMIC CYCLES

In both men and women the orgasmic cycle is much the same. During the excitement and plateau phases the sexual organs fill with blood; in women the clitoris becomes prominent and the vagina and vulva swell; and in men the penis becomes erect. Orgasm is characterized by muscular contractions; the body then returns to its nonaroused state.

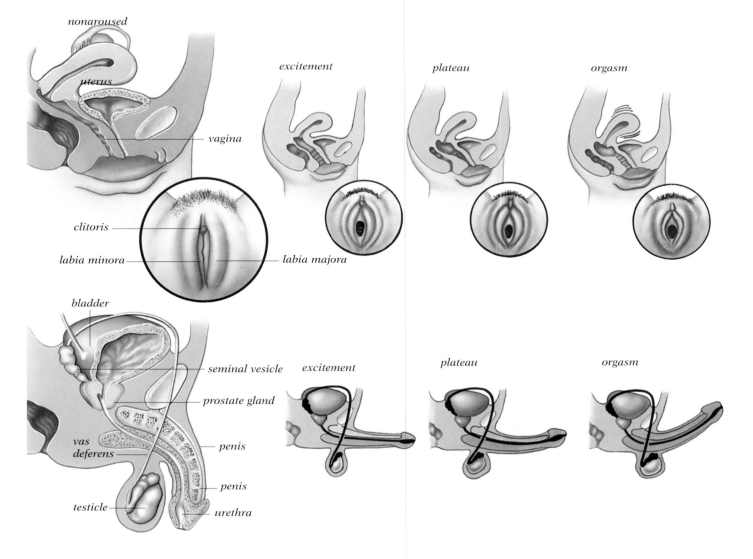

I just can't bear to tell my doctor about my sexual problems; I feel so embarrassed. What shall I do about it?

You don't have to tell him or her everything. Just explain that you have a problem in your sex life, and ask to be referred to a specialist counselor.

Are there times when sex problems are more likely?

Adolescence, pregnancy, and the so-called midlife crisis are all stressful periods that can produce sexual difficulties. Menopause produces less problems than may be expected, and a late flowering of sexuality can often occur as a happy bonus in middle age.

Can sexual problems masquerade as some other form of trouble?

Sometimes this happens. The old joke about "Not tonight, I've got a headache" can be very real. However, now that sex is no longer such a taboo subject, problems appear in their direct form much more than they used to.

I was talking to a very close friend the other day about my sex life, and she appeared to be horrified at some of the things I said my husband and I did. Are we deviant or is my friend unadventurous?

This raises a complicated issue: what is normal and what isn't? The answer is that there is no single definition of normality. What is acceptable and mutually enjoyable for some couples is not for others. Whether or not a couple wish to experiment is up to them. However, there are some basic ideas worth considering. For instance, never try anything that may be physically dangerous, and avoid practices that are degrading, demeaning, or humiliating to one or both partners. Apart from that, though, there is a wide range of sexual practices that can be extremely rewarding and satisfying to both partners.

Alcohol can have a detrimental effect on a man's sexual performance because it has a depressing effect on the nervous system. One drink too many may mean there will be difficulty in achieving an erection; and alcoholism may cause long-term problems, such as loss of libido (see Alcoholism).

Drugs prescribed for the treatment of depression or circulatory diseases can also affect sexual response. Erection may be possible, but there may not be an orgasm, and there may be little interest in sex at all. Any man receiving medical treatment who has sexual problems should consult his doctor about the possible side effects.

Hormone deficiency can cause loss of libido, but this is very rare. It can be due to a low level of testosterone, which is a male hormone. Men with this condition are likely to have little interest in sex, and hardly, if ever, masturbate. Hormone replacement therapy is possible, but it does not have a very high success rate (see Masturbation; Testosterone).

Although there are many problems relating to the physical side of sex, by far the greatest number of sexual problems are psychological.

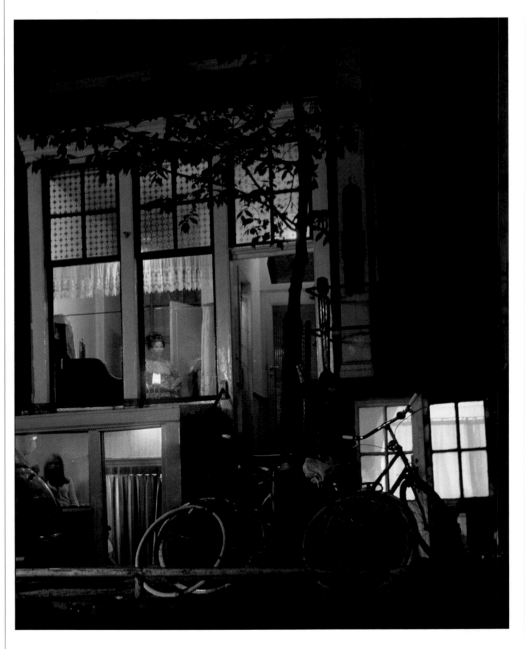

▲ *A brothel in Amsterdam, Netherlands. For some people prostitutes offer the only outlet for their sexual needs.*

Sexual knowledge is much more openly available to young people nowadays, and adult discussion of sexual matters is more free and easy than was once the case. In spite of this, many of the old problems remain for some people.

Psychological problems

Virtually every case concerning sexual problems or feelings of inadequacy is caused by anxiety, which can arise for a number of reasons (see Anxiety).

Religious views: Strict religious beliefs taught in childhood may interfere with a person's sexual happiness, even if he or she has ceased to regard those beliefs as truth. Most religious texts contain guides to moral behavior, but it is only too easy for these to be carried to the extreme by a religiously zealous person. Some beliefs can make sexual happiness extremely difficult, either by preventing sexual activity directly or by producing enormous sexual guilt that is hard to get rid of.

Sexual shock: Strong sexual fears lasting for many years can also be produced by some frightening or degrading sexual experience in early life. Child assault, rape, and catching sexually transmitted

▼ *Sex is an all-pervasive influence in modern life, and is used to advertise such commodities as cars, perfume, and clothes.*

diseases are all examples of experiences that can affect a person's sexual activity and beliefs later in life.

Poor sex education: Although sex education is now easily available to those who seek it, the taboos that surround the subject still exist. Many parents still find it difficult to discuss sexual matters with their children. Surveys have shown that in adolescence children would rather talk to an older friend than to a parent.

Alcohol: Although too much alcohol can produce a temporary inability to reach a climax in men, the real danger lies when an individual does not realize that alcohol is the reason for his temporary incapacity. He may brood over his weakness; then anger and fear may build up; and after a number of such failures he may become psychologically impotent.

Parental models: Parents inevitably transmit to their children not only facts but attitudes about sex. They do this not only directly but also by their own behavior, and if negative or fearful attitudes are shown by parents, these attitudes are likely to be reflected in the children and can produce difficulties when those children grow up.

Male problems

Male psychological problems are of two types. The first is concerned with performance, and here the man becomes very anxious about his ability to make love satisfactorily. He may worry whether his

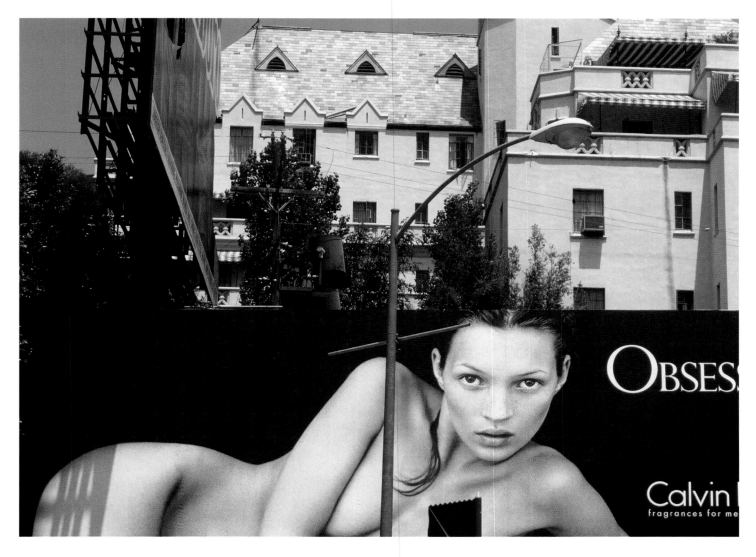

partner will find him attractive enough, or whether he can satisfy her and make her happy. He may worry about his potency and the possibility that he might reach orgasm too soon.

Problems of this first type include: impotence, in which the male is unable to achieve an erection sufficient for intercourse, even though he may have been able to do so at least once in the past (see Impotence); premature ejaculation, in which the man is unable to delay or control his orgasm; and ejaculatory specificity, a very rare disability in which a man cannot ejaculate within his partner's vagina but has no difficulty with erection or ejaculation while masturbating. It is important to remember, however, that virtually every man suffers from occasional bouts of impotence or occasional premature ejaculation, and usually this should not be a cause for any concern. It is only when such difficulties occur repeatedly that treatment should be considered as an option.

Acceptability problems

The second type of male problem has to do with the acceptability (or unacceptability) to his partner of the type of sexual pattern that he might enjoy. Problems arise because some men very often have surprisingly specific likings within their sex lives. Men frequently have fantasies which they like to think of or play out while lovemaking, and some of these may seem to have little relation for the partner to either the act of sex or to the warm and intimate relationship that society seems in general to regard as its natural accompaniment.

The impact of a male's desires, and awareness of his sometimes strange fantasies, can often produce distaste and fear in a woman. Equally, a man who is aware of this possibility may himself experience fear, which can prevent him from relaxing during lovemaking and also render him sexually inadequate.

Female problems

As with males, female psychosexual problems are of two types. The first manifests itself as physical difficulty in making love when the cause is not actually physical, so that intercourse becomes painful or impossible; the cause is emotional and due to sexual anxiety.

The worries are not about adequacy of performance but are concerned with sexual fear. Fear of an unwanted pregnancy, fear of being hurt, fear of being used or abused or being regarded merely as a sex object, fear of being abandoned, and fear of being thought of badly by others can affect women deeply. These fears may be manifested as general sexual dysfunction, in which the woman does

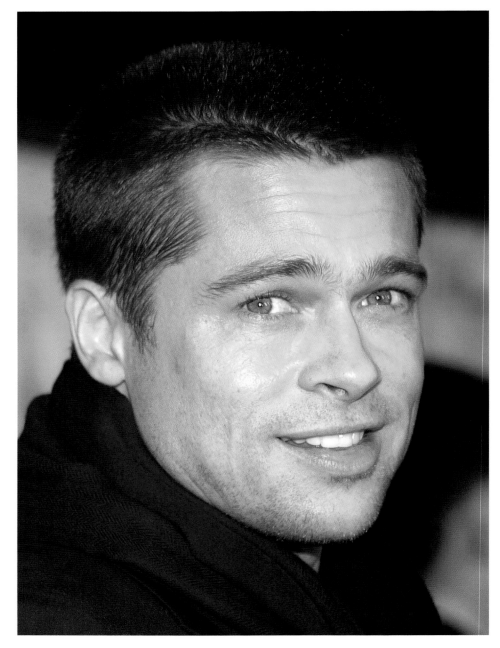

▲ *Brad Pitt is an example of a male movie star who is considered a sex symbol; many women find him sexually attractive and men may view him as a sexual role model.*

not respond to erotic stimulation and does not experience the excitement phase of the sexual cycle. It used to be commonplace to refer to this condition as frigidity.

Alternatively, anxiety may produce anorgasmia, in which, though arousal takes place normally, orgasm is never reached. Some women are content to remain at a high level of arousal for a satisfying period without having an orgasm. To most women, however, this can be a very frustrating and intolerable experience.

"Dyspareunia" is the formal term for excessively painful or difficult intercourse. It may, of course, result from poor arousal technique by the man or from physical causes such as infection or internal injury, but more often it arises as a result of sexual anxiety. One particular form of dyspareunia is vaginismus. In this condition,

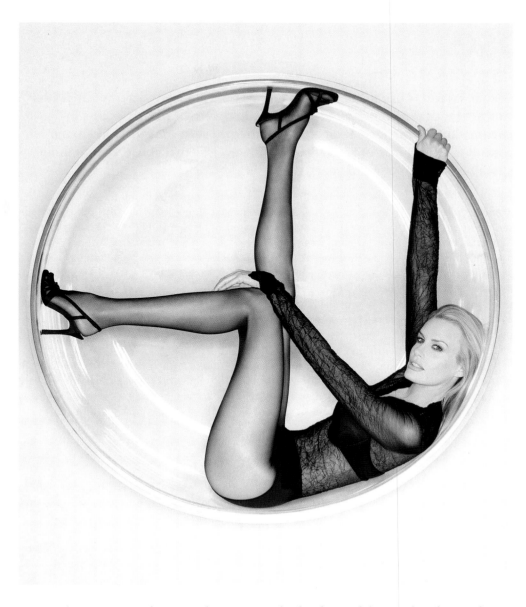

have created problems for others. To be sexually assertive, to take the leading role, or to demand instead of merely accepting seems threatening to some women and can produce anxiety and fear instead of excitement and pleasure. When such worries are present, sexual happiness can be impaired.

Treatment

Although specific problems such as premature ejaculation and vaginismus can be treated by well-established physical methods, nearly all sex therapy for either sex takes the form of specialist counseling together with a definite program of events designed to restore a full and fulfilling sexual life. Published estimates suggest that at least 50 percent of couples experience some kind of sexual problem at some stage in their relationship; couples should therefore feel no shame about attending sex therapy.

Except when a client has no stable sexual relationship, sex therapists know that sexual problems almost always concern the partner of that person as well, and both partners must thus be prepared to be involved in the therapy. Group therapy is also used.

Clients for sex therapy are often unaware of basic aspects of sexual physiology and techniques. Sex education helps reduce the fear of the unknown in sex and reduces anxiety.

Therapists try to counter negative attitudes toward sex and help clients to be happy about seeking and accepting the sexual pleasure they have previously denied themselves.

▲ *Overtly suggestive advertising keeps sex at the forefront of the mind and may play a part in desires and expectations of sexuality.*

the outer third of the vaginal tube becomes prone to strong and uncontrollable contractions, virtually closing off the vaginal entrance. Vaginismus most often occurs in women who are afraid that intercourse will be painful. In some women a contributing factor may be guilt and fear that have arisen due to poor sexual education, repressive upbringing, or some kind of sexual trauma. The condition is most often treated by the use of graded dilators which the woman introduces into her vagina over a series of treatment sessions. Eventually, the woman will become confident enough to attempt sexual intercourse.

Attitude problems

The second type of female problem arises from the radical changes in sexual expectations that women are now undergoing. The realization that orgasm is as much their right as it is for men, and that they have as much right to a rich and full sexual life as the male does, may have come as a liberation to many women but seems to

Sexual preferences

Attraction and desire can be felt for people of the opposite sex or for the same sex (see Homosexuality). Sometimes people have equally strong desires for people of the same and the opposite sex. This is called bisexuality. Just what it is that attracts people to each other is not known. Physical factors are also important with regard to attraction and desire—whether someone is attractive to look at, and whether he or she looks interesting. Psychological factors are also important; people may choose a potential partner because of his or her likeness to, or differences from, a mother or father with whom they have had a good or bad relationship, for example.

Long-lasting and happy relationships cannot be built on sexual attraction alone. They come from sharing experiences, understanding the other person, and working together to build up friendship as well as a good sexual partnership.

See also: **Sexual dysfunction**

Sexual abuse

Questions and Answers

I am a teacher. What should I do if I think one of my pupils is being sexually abused at home?

You must approach someone who is professionally trained to handle this type of situation; your school probably has guidelines and your principal will know about them. Perhaps there is a therapist or counselor already attached to the school. Ignoring a situation where sexual abuse is taking place can have serious consequences; however, false accusations can be extremely damaging to the alleged assailant. The type of case you describe must be handled by experienced individuals with extreme care and sensitively.

Can a person suffer sexual abuse that is not physical? I think my sister might be being abused by her boyfriend in this way.

Many therapists agree that if a person is continually subject to verbal abuse and comments that make him or her feel threatened or degraded sexually—for example, if your sister's partner makes demeaning and critical sexual remarks, using sexual names or making her feel she has to engage in unwanted sexual acts—then this is a type of sexual abuse. Your sister should seek help; it could be that she needs to get out of this relationship.

I was sexually abused by my stepfather from the age of 11 until I left home at 16. I never told anyone. I am now 23, and have never had a boyfriend; I find it difficult to trust people and to form friendships. What can I do?

You need professional help so that you can accept what has happened, recover fully, and move on. If there is a doctor you know and trust, visit him or her for advice and a referral to a good therapist or counselor.

Sexual assault is usually defined as any sexual contact or attempt at sexual contact that takes place without the victim's consent or that occurs in circumstances where a person is unable to give such consent. Any sexual assault is an instance of sexual abuse; however, sexual abuse is commonly sustained over a period of years.

Many people associate the term "sexual abuse" with sexual relations that take place between family members, such as between parents and children, or brothers and sisters; however, sexual abuse can take place outside a family as well.

Abuse is a misuse of power; sexual abuse might involve marital rape, nonconsensual incest, sexual verbal or physical harassment, child molestation, sexual touching—any kind of sexual relations that involve coercion, force, or intimidation, or when the victim is not in a position to give consent (for example; if he or she is a minor, has been drugged, or is too drunk or intoxicated to know what is happening). However, because abuse, as opposed to assault, usually takes place over a period of time, it almost invariably involves attack by someone the victim knows, such as a family member, partner, friend, colleague, or friend of the family.

Sexual abuse is common, but the figures sometimes quoted—such as that more than one in four girls and one in six boys in the United States have suffered such abuse by the time they are 18 years old—might call into question exactly what is meant in many of these cases by "sexual abuse." An exact definition is key in this respect.

Causes

By definition, victims of sexual abuse do not cause or invite the abuse to take place. Only the person initiating the sexual contact or harassment is responsible.

A perpetrator of certain forms of sexual abuse—for example, rape—is thought to abuse primarily out of anger, out of a need to feel powerful. Because he (or, very occasionally, she) wishes to control or dominate the victim, control and domination may be the sole motive (see Rape).

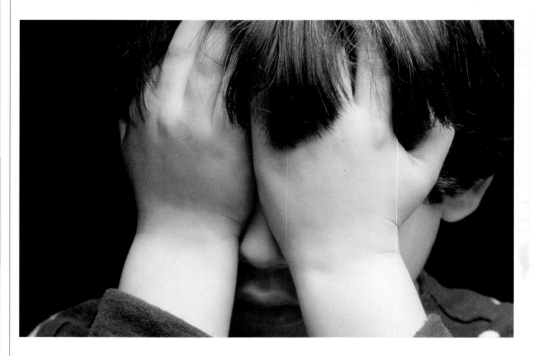

▲ *A child who has been sexually abused will be unhappy, lack confidence, and feel general depression and despair.*

Figures suggest that about a third of sex offenders have been abused themselves—in terms of sexual abuse, physical abuse, or emotional neglect—by one or both parents, by primary caregivers, or by some kind of authority figure before the age of 16 years. The abuser was often someone other than their parents. About 60 percent of those abused had been separated from their biological parents as children. Many sex offenders have a history of drug and alcohol abuse (see Drug Abuse).

Symptoms of abuse; stages of recovery

A victim of a serious sexual assault, such as rape, initially experiences shock; this might be emotional as well as physical, and could be expressed in a controlled or withdrawn manner, or it might be extremely expressive, including crying, screaming, or shaking.

He or she will probably have trouble communicating to others what has happened. Estimates suggest that only about a third of victims of a sexual assault actually report it to the authorities, either at the time of the attack or later on.

A victim of rape or of some other form of serious sexual abuse is then likely to go through a stage of denial. He or she may try to carry on life normally, in an attempt to forget about what has happened or—when the abuse is sustained over time—what is continuing to happen. This is an attempt to deal with the confusion and turmoil he or she is feeling. Victims of sexual abuse may also attempt to convince themselves that the assault did not really take place; or if it did, that it is unlikely to happen again.

At a later stage the victim often reexperiences his or her initial feelings of

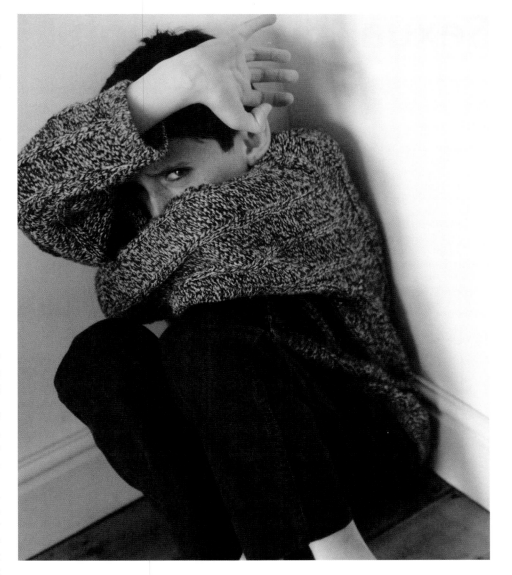

▲ *In a vulnerable young person, systematic abuse instills fear and a distrust of people. These feelings can be overcome with therapy.*

shock; such feelings are usually triggered by memories of the assault itself. Feelings of depression, anxiety, and shame often become worse around this time. Later still, the victim of a serious assault often comes to experience intense feelings of anger, often toward him- or herself, his or her friends or family, a partner, society, the legal system, or all men or women.

Other symptoms that may occur after any form of sexual abuse include sleeplessness, nightmares, flashbacks, a sense of vulnerability and loss of self-confidence, mistrust of others, fear of being alone, overeating or loss of appetite, feelings of grief and despair, and stress-related illnesses and complaints (see Depression).

Treatment and outlook

Clearly the first step in a person's recovery from sexual abuse involves removal of the source of that abuse. Often such a situation must be handled with extreme sensitivity, particularly when the abuser is a family member. In some circumstances, it is the victim who must leave or be removed from the situation where he or she is being abused. Apart from treatment for physical symptoms, anyone who has suffered serious sexual abuse over a prolonged period will almost certainly require professional counseling and therapy (see Sexually Transmitted Diseases).

The emotions and physical symptoms that the victim experiences are seen by many therapists as part of the natural process of coming to terms with what has happened and moving toward recovery. With skillful support and therapy, a victim of abuse can eventually overcome feelings of despair and vulnerability, and can learn to direct feelings of anger and blame toward the assailant.

The final stage in the recovery from the assault is what is termed "integration," or "closure." As the victim integrates the thoughts and feelings stemming from the abuse into his or her life experience, he or she begins to be able to cope.

With support, education, and time, the victim should eventually feel able to carry on with his or her life.

See also: **Child abuse; Incest**

Sexual dysfunction

Sexual dysfunction, whether experienced by men or women, can disrupt personal relationships and cause profound distress. Although a sexual problem may have physical causes, anxiety can make the problem worse.

Sexual relationships are important and, when serious and long-lasting, may be a source of much happiness and life enhancement. But such relationships are never simple, and there is much that can go wrong, on a physical and a psychological level. Everyone should have some knowledge of the causes and treatment of failure to achieve satisfactory sex. Although the physical aspects of such problems can be divided into male and female causes, sexual dysfunction must always be considered as a problem involving both partners. Many sexual difficulties are psychosomatic because a sexual relationship involves, or should involve, strong emotions and other mental factors that can lead to problems. These include ignorance, faulty expectations and myths derived from the media, poor ability to communicate, and undue concern over social factors.

Male dysfunction

The most common form of male sexual dysfunction is the inability to achieve or sustain a sufficiently firm erection to allow normal vaginal sexual intercourse. This is called impotence, and it is a cause of great distress to many males. The distress arises not only because it prevents the enjoyment of sex but also because it is regarded by many males as an indication of lack of masculinity. This view is, in itself, a common cause of impotence.

Almost all sexually experienced men have suffered episodes of impotence, and these are almost always of purely psychological origin. Only a very small proportion are due to organic disease, and such cases usually involve older men. Psychogenic impotence is often due to anxiety about performance and may be about the attitude of the partner. Fortunately, most women regard occasional episodes of impotence as unimportant, calling for sympathy and understanding rather than criticism, and in no way reflecting on the man's masculinity. Organic impotence can often be helped by drugs such as Viagra.

Premature ejaculation is the condition in which the male orgasm occurs at such an early stage in sexual intercourse as to deprive both partners of satisfaction. Sometimes this occurs even before penetration. The majority of cases of premature ejaculation are due to the excessive excitement often occurring in inexperienced men. This can be relied on to settle in due course.

Priapism is a rare disorder in which a firm erection fails to subside after an orgasm. This is potentially dangerous because after about four hours, the blood in the penis is likely to clot and then to form damaging internal scar tissue. It is important to seek immediate medical attention for this condition. The treatment is to drain the blood from the erectile tissue through a wide-bore needle inserted under anesthesia. Priapism has been known to be caused by drug abuse.

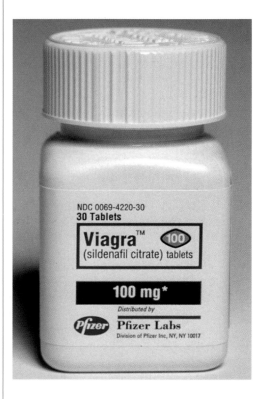

▲ *The introduction of Viagra, a drug to help cure erectile dysfunction, revealed the prevalence of the problem in the United States.*

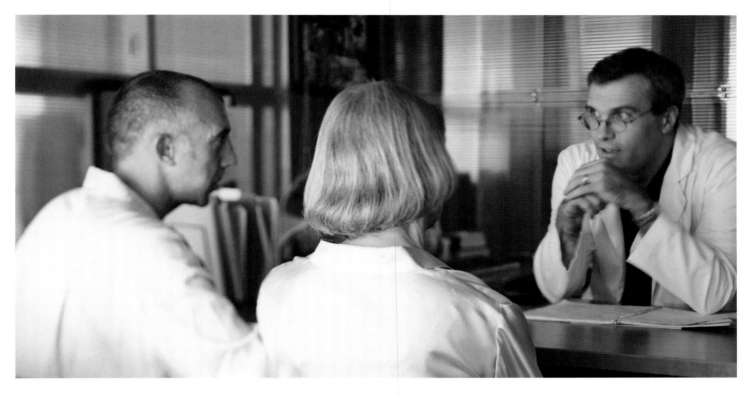

▲ *Partners who are experiencing sexual problems may find that a sex therapist can help resolve them. A therapist can assist in improving communication between partners and will help to identify specific problems.*

Peyronie's disease is a disorder of the penis, of unknown origin, in which local thickening and rigidity of the fibrous tissue sheath of the organ results in a sharp bend in the penis when it is erect. This may interfere with sexual intercourse and cause discomfort to both partners, or may even prevent normal intercourse. The condition may be helped by a course of steroid injections, but surgical removal of the thickened areas is often required.

Female dysfunction

Failure to achieve orgasm in women is often described as frigidity by men disappointed in their expectations of arousing desire and an enthusiastic sexual response in their partners. It may be the result of lack of affection, or of its expression, by the man, or of his lack of sexual understanding and technique. However, there are other possible causes, including recent childbirth, pain during intercourse, fear of pregnancy, trauma following rape, or the use of drugs to treat insomnia, high blood pressure, or depression. About 10 percent of all women will never experience orgasm, and about 50 percent never experience orgasm during intercourse. This is usually due to insufficient stimulation, but it is often regarded by the man as a criticism of his masculinity.

Other problems

The medical term for painful sexual intercourse is dyspareunia. This may have many causes, both physical and psychological. Physical causes include vaginal or uterine infection, vaginal scars from stitching after childbirth (episiotomy repair), or rare congenital vaginal defects. Pain can also be psychological, however, and is often experienced as an expression of fear or anger, or as an unconscious strategy to avoid unwanted sex. An extreme condition of seemingly involuntary rejection of attempted sexual intercourse is called vaginismus. This condition is very difficult to treat. Many who suffer from the conditions mentioned here could benefit by visiting their family doctor to discuss treatment options and referrals to specialists. Although sex is the means of reproducing, it is also much more than that. Sexual emotions, including attraction, desire, and love, are among the strongest and most exciting feelings that people experience. Sexual interest in other people does not usually begin until adolescence. At this time, many boys and girls find themselves strongly attracted to others of their own sex. Most of them grow out of this phase, and their interest focuses on someone of the opposite sex.

Some couples are afraid to communicate their sexual needs, desires, and preferences to each other for fear of being rejected or despised. Therapy can help them overcome this fear and avoid any rejection that otherwise might have occurred.

The direct methods of reducing anxiety that are commonly used in behavior therapy can effectively be used where sexual anxiety is concerned. For example, a fear of intercourse can be reduced by teaching people to enjoy general body sensuality without intercourse, as in sensate focusing (see Behavior Therapy).

Although the idea of a set program of changes in behavior may seem strange, a therapist often will prescribe changes in behavior in a graduated series of sexual activities to encourage a couple's enjoyment of body contact and sexual versatility. Such a program helps to overcome the shyness that some couples still feel even after years of being together.

See also: **Drug abuse; Hormones; Penis and disorders; Psychology; Sex; Therapy**

Sexually transmitted diseases

Sexually transmitted diseases (STDs) are infections that are contracted during sexual activity. Early diagnosis and prompt treatment with appropriate drugs are essential to avoid side effects such as infertility.

Sexually transmitted disease is in fact not a single disease but a collection of several different conditions that are grouped together because they are all acquired as a result of sexual intercourse with a person who has the infection. AIDS is a condition caused by the complex HIV virus that is, among other ways, sexually transmitted. Research into HIV and AIDS is extensive, and while some progress has been made, there is still no cure for what is usually a fatal condition. Syphilis, gonorrhea, genital warts, chlamydial infection, and genital herpes are prone to complications, some of which can be very serious; less serious sexually transmitted diseases include trichomoniasis, monilia, and pubic lice (see Lice; Trichomoniasis).

HIV and AIDS

Acquired immunodeficiency syndrome (AIDS) is the most serious of the sexually transmitted diseases. Since the first official AIDS cases were reported in 1981, about 22 million people had died of the disease worldwide by 2001; about 400,000 of these deaths were in the United States.

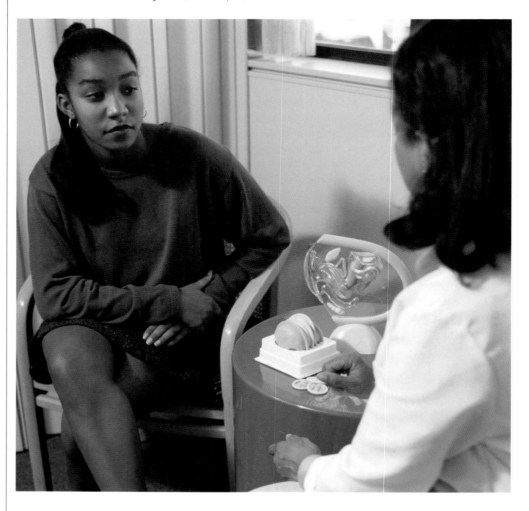

▲ *Young people are particularly at risk when it comes to sexually transmitted diseases because of greater sexual freedom at an increasingly earlier age.*

AIDS is caused by the human immunodeficiency virus (HIV), which is usually acquired during sexual contact through the blood, vaginal fluid, or semen. It can also be transmitted through infected needles or blood transfusions, or from an infected mother to her child through the blood or breast milk. When a person is infected with HIV, the body makes special antibodies to try to fight the virus off. A person is diagnosed as having HIV when a blood test finds these antibodies in the blood; the person is then said to be HIV-positive. In 2003, about 800,000 to 900,000 people were HIV-positive.

HIV slowly wears down the immune system, reducing the number of helper T lymphocyte cells, also called T4 cells, that help fight off infections (see Immune System). When an HIV-positive person has less than 200 T4 cells, he or she has developed AIDS (the average healthy person has 500 to 1,500 T4 cells in 1 ml of blood). About 300,000 people were living with AIDS in the United States in 2003.

The development from HIV to AIDS may happen quickly or take 10 or more years. Symptoms of HIV include fevers, night sweats, diarrhea, and swollen lymph nodes. AIDS-related symptoms include severe weight loss and brain tumors. Once AIDS has developed, opportunistic infections occur—most commonly, pneumocystis pneumonia; a skin cancer called Kaposi's sarcoma; cytomegalovirus, which affects the eyes; and candida (see Thrush)—until one or a combination of such infections proves fatal (see Opportunistic Infection).

There is no cure for HIV or AIDS. Drug treatment with highly active antiretroviral therapy (HAART) given to people who are HIV-positive has decreased the death rate from AIDS. However, HAART has to be taken for the rest of the patient's life to be effective and some patients have such severe side effects that they are unable to take it.

Syphilis

Syphilis is considered one of the more serious sexually transmitted infections because it is likely to result, if untreated, in permanent disability or even death. The bacteria are spread from one person to another during intercourse. They can also be passed from an infected mother to her child during pregnancy; therefore the baby may be born with congenital syphilis. Routine blood testing of all expectant mothers and the treatment of those found to be infected have made congenital syphilis a rare condition.

The incubation period of syphilis varies widely, as do the symptoms of the first or primary stage of the disease. This makes for enormous difficulty in the early recognition of the disease, which is essential for a total and permanent cure to be achieved.

An indication of syphilis is a single painless ulcer (chancre) appearing where the germ has entered the body; in or around the genitals, anus, or mouth (see Ulcers). The ulcer heals by itself, and because of this, many people fail to consult a doctor. An added complication is that sometimes a chancre does not appear at all. For this reason, it is essential for anyone who thinks that he or she may have been in contact with a sexually transmitted disease to seek advice from a doctor or treatment center, because a cure can be guaranteed only if treatment is given in the early stages of the disease.

Gonorrhea

Gonorrhea is another bacterial disease that is very common. It is contracted by sexual intercourse with an infected person. About 80 percent of infected women have no symptoms and are generally unaware that they have it. Some have pain passing urine (dysuria) or cystitis and some develop lower abdominal pain from infection of the fallopian tubes (see Salpingitis), which can lead to pelvic inflammatory disease and subsequent sterility. Diagnosis is not easy; it is best carried out by a doctor or treatment center. It consists of finding the bacteria in specimens obtained during a vaginal examination. In men inflammation of the testes can occur. In less than a week after being infected, pain on passing urine develops, followed by a profuse discharge of pus from the opening at the end of the penis, the urinary meatus. The diagnosis of gonorrhea is confirmed by discovering bacteria in the discharge.

Treatment in both sexes is usually by a single dose of penicillin, given either as an injection or as capsules; abstention from

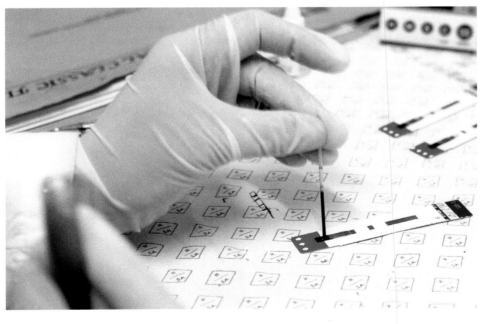

▲ *Blood samples of pregnant women are tested for HIV in a clinic in Soweto, South Africa. Sexually transmitted diseases are particularly dangerous for pregnant women, since they can pass the diseases to their babies, which can, in some cases, endanger the babies' lives.*

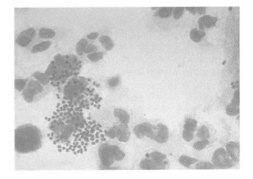

▲ *Diagnosis of gonorrhea is made by microscopic examination, which reveals the presence of the bacteria* Neisseria gonorrhoeae *in the specimen. This is taken from the vagina or, in men, from urinary discharge.*

Questions and Answers

Can an STD make it more difficult to get pregnant?

Yes. STDs are more likely to cause permanent damage in women than in men. One of the most serious ways they can affect women is to make them sterile because the tube down which the monthly egg or ovum passes becomes blocked due to disease.

Does either urinating or taking a shower after sexual intercourse have any effect in reducing the risk of getting an STD?

Washing the sexual parts thoroughly with soap and water and passing urine after sex can reduce the risk of catching a sexually transmitted disease, especially in men, but they do not eliminate the risk. Using a condom offers a much greater degree of protection.

Can one become immune to STDs?

Unlike diseases such as measles, an attack of one of the sexually transmitted diseases does not protect against future attacks. Sexually transmitted diseases can be caught many times, and people do not generally become immune to them.

Can STD affect an unborn baby in the womb?

Yes. Syphilis may cause stillbirth, miscarriage, deformities, or even death of the baby after birth. Therefore all expectant mothers have blood tests for syphilis during pregnancy; if they test positive, treatment can be given to protect the baby. Genital herpes can also be fatal if passed by a woman to her baby during childbirth; if there are open vesicles at the time of birth, the baby will be delivered by cesarean section. Gonorrhea and chlamydia can affect a baby's eyes if the bacteria are active when the baby is born. AIDS can be transmitted before birth from an infected mother to her baby.

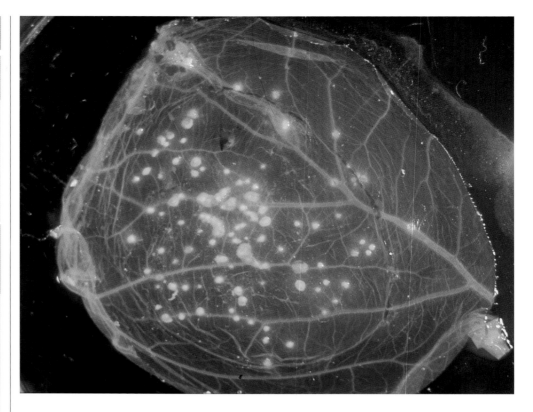

▲ *A microscopic view of the genital herpes virus, which causes painful blisters. There is no cure, and genital herpes has reached epidemic proportions in the United States.*

alcohol and sexual intercourse for several weeks is also important. The relief of symptoms after treatment is dramatic, but supervision must be maintained to ensure that the cure is permanent and complete. An attack of gonorrhea confers no immunity for the future. Patients should ensure that all those with whom they have recently had sexual contact are made aware of the facts and go for examination. The use of a condom during intercourse gives considerable protection to both partners. Gonorrhea is not hereditary, but a gonococcal infection can be passed on to babies and young girls, either during birth or by close contact with an infected mother.

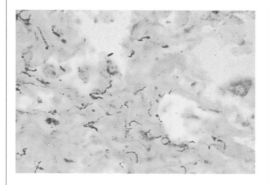

▲ *Syphilis is an infection caused by the* bacterium Treponema pallidum. *The characteristic threadlike spiral cells of the bacteria are visible.*

► *Syphilis sufferers may also develop a papular rash, characterized by small, solid elevations of the skin, that appears on the palms of the hands and the soles of the feet.*

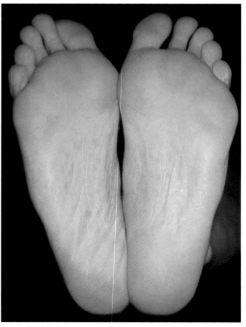

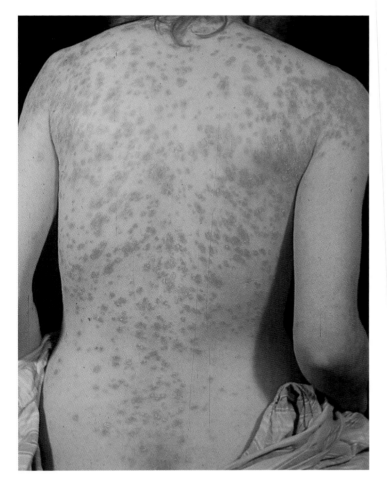

◄ Unless treated immediately, syphilis will move into its secondary stage with the development of a roseolar skin rash, affecting the trunk and limbs, that can vary greatly in type and intensity. Left untreated, the rash eventually fades and the disease enters the dormant stage.

both. PID is a serious condition that may cause severe and persistent pelvic pain and commonly leads to female infertility.

Genital herpes

Genital herpes is a sexually transmitted disease that has reached epidemic proportions in the United States. The main problem is that, being a virus, herpes cannot be cured and so each new sufferer adds to the pool of carriers. There are two types of herpes simplex virus, both of which cause painful blisters (vesicles), localized swelling, and sometimes fever. HSV 1 was at one time mainly found around the mouth (cold sores), but possibly as a result of widespread oral sexual practices, HSV 1 is now the most common cause of genital herpes. HSV 2 is spread by sexual contact and the blisters can be found in and around the genitals, around the anus, and on the bladder, buttocks, thighs, and legs of both sexes. This condition exists in two states: latent and active. After the first attack, the virus travels up a local sensory nerve and then lies dormant in the body. It waits until an attack is triggered, then emerges again, usually in the same spot time and time again, as a painful blister. During latent periods when no blisters are open, sexual partners will not catch herpes from the carrier, but the carrier is extremely contagious when blisters are open. It is possible that the carrier will be unaware of their existence if the vesicles are inside the vagina, on the cervix, or in the urethra. Attacks appear to be linked to physical and emotional low points, such as during times of depression or stress, illness, just before a period, or during bad weather, or to local stimulation of the affected areas.

Genital herpes is painful and depressing to an adult, and it is often fatal if it is passed by a pregnant sufferer to her baby as the baby passes down the birth canal. A pregnant woman who has suffered genital herpes, even if she has not had an attack for some time, should always tell the medical team about her condition. They will monitor her during the pregnancy (see Pregnancy) and, if there are open vesicles at the time of birth, the baby can be saved if delivered by cesarean section (see Cesarean Birth).

Because a virus is entwined with the cells of the host, and anything that harms the virus invariably harms the host, genital herpes cannot yet be cured, but there are ways of speeding up the recovery time from attacks and making them less unpleasant. Keeping the affected areas clean and dry will stop secondary infection. Salt baths and cold compresses will ease pain. Staying free of stress and healthy will help the body erect defenses against attacks. In most cases attacks will come most months for the first year and gradually tail off, becoming less frequent as the years go by.

Although there is no cure for herpes, the severity and frequency of relapses of the disease can be markedly reduced by means of the drug aciclovir (Zovirax) taken by mouth. Since genital herpes has been linked to cancer of the cervix, women sufferers should have regular Pap smears at least once a year (see Pap Smear).

Genital warts

It has been known for some time that sexually promiscuous women are much more likely than those in single relationships to develop

NSU

What was once called nonspecific urethritis (NSU) is now known to be caused by germs called *Chlamydia trachomatis*. The number of cases continues to increase at a rapid rate, making chlamydial infection more common than all the other sexually transmitted diseases together. Chlamydial germs are very much smaller than most bacteria and can survive only inside cells. It is for this reason that the cause of what was called nonspecific urethritis took so long to be established. Some cases get better quickly and present no problem, but in other cases recurrences are common. Chlamydial STD in males is urethritis or inflammation of the urethra that is now clearly distinguished from the other main cause of urethritis, which is gonorrhea. Since the treatment, management, and implications of gonorrhea and chlamydial infection are quite different, when a specialist suspects chlamydial infection, he or she will make sure, by means of microscopic examination and laboratory tests of the discharge, that it is not in fact a mild case of gonorrhea. The main symptom is a discharge from the tip of the penis. The discharge is usually clear white to gray in color, not the creamy yellow matter that is characteristic of gonorrhea, and it is similar to semen in appearance. The quantity varies a great deal but is usually a small amount, sometimes no more than a moistness at the tip of the penis. The second common symptom is pain on passing urine, the severity of which is extremely variable. Often there is no pain at all or there is just irritation.

Chlamydial infection in women may, like gonorrhea, initially be symptomless, but almost all cases of chronic pelvic inflammatory disease (PID) are caused by chlamydial infection or gonorrhea or

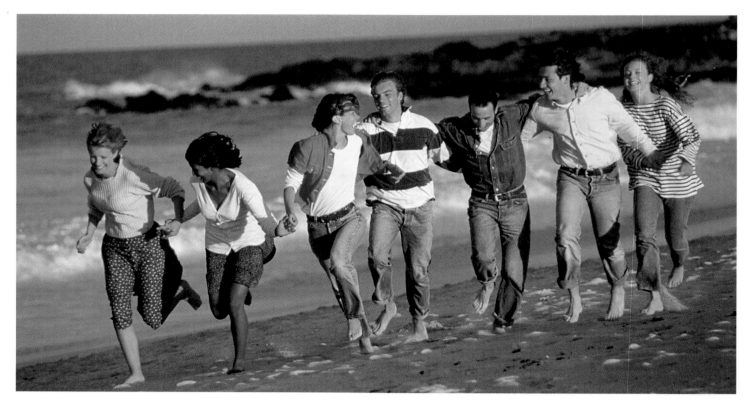

▲ *Young adults under the age of 25 are at the highest risk of being infected with STDs.*

cancer of the cervix. The link is now known not to be genital herpes but genital warts, which are commonly transmitted sexually. The virus that causes genital warts is the human papilloma virus and it is this virus that contributes to the causation of cervical cancer. The recent development of a vaccine against genital warts gives hope that a reduction can be achieved in the prevalence of this very common female cancer (see Cervix and Cervical Smears).

Identifying discharges

Women often worry that vaginal discharge or a change in what is normal for them may mean that they have caught an STD. However, although a vaginal discharge should not be dismissed as trivial, and tests and treatment may be required, many discharges are in fact normal, and only a few are caused by a serious condition. The quantity of the discharge, which is often what gives rise to alarm, can vary widely from one woman to another and is particularly likely to increase in certain situations. What is important, in relation to the possibility of infection or other disease, is not the quantity but the quality or type of discharge (see Vaginal Discharge).

Clear mucous discharges are unlikely to be caused by disease, but a discharge that is discolored, causes soreness or irritation of the vagina or vulva, or has an unpleasant odor is much more likely to be related to infection of the female genital organs. A thin, yellow discharge is suggestive of trichomonas infection; a thick, white discharge is characteristic of thrush (monilia); and brown discharges are decomposed blood, which is an indication of internal bleeding. This is most likely to be due to erosion or ulceration of the neck of the womb or cervix, but it can be caused by cancer of the womb and must therefore always be investigated.

If an unpleasant discharge continues for more than a week, a doctor should be consulted or a woman should attend a special clinic without delay, especially if it is accompanied by fever or abdominal pain, if there is a possibility of STD, if the discharge is bloodstained or brown and a menstrual period is not due, if it is accompanied by pain on passing urine, if there is soreness and irritation with discharge, or if it has an unpleasant odor. A doctor will ask about the type of discharge and recent sexual relationships. He or she will probably examine the vagina with a gloved hand and with a plastic or metal instrument, using a light to see inside. He or she may take specimens from the vagina and neck of the womb and possibly also from the urethra and rectum for laboratory analysis.

STDs and young adults

According to a 2004 report, half of all young Americans will get a sexually transmitted disease by the age of 25. Genital warts, chlamydia, and trichomoniasis account for 88 percent of all the new cases of STDs. Teenagers 15 years and older who have had sex have the highest STD rates of any age group in the country. The reason for this large number of cases may be attributed to the development of new contraceptives since the 1960s, which has led to an alteration in attitudes and habits in sexual behavior and, consequently, greater sexual freedom at an earlier age. However, a more open approach to sex demands a need for more awareness and thoughtfulness toward one's partner, rather than less. Young people can suffer from ignorance or embarrassment about asking about methods of protecting themselves from sexually transmitted diseases.

Prevention

Several precautions can be taken to reduce the chances of getting a sexually transmitted disease. Abstinence and avoiding sex with more than one person can reduce the risk. Condoms and a

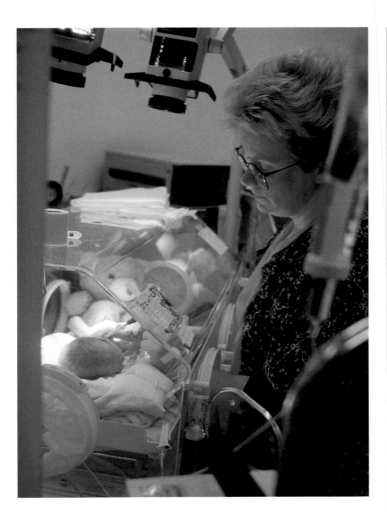

▲ *Sexually transmitted diseases can have tragic consequences for a baby born to an infected mother. The baby may suffer from jaundice, anemia, a swollen liver and spleen, fever, and skin rashes and sores. Even worse, some babies with syphilis are stillborn, or die soon after birth.*

spermicide should be used for sexual intercourse of any kind (see Contraception). Using a condom will give both partners a considerable degree of protection against all forms of STD. Water-based lubricants should be used rather than oil-based lubricants, which damage rubber. For both the man and the woman a thorough cleansing of the genital area with soap and water before and after intercourse will kill a large proportion of the bacteria with which they may have been contaminated. For men, if they pass urine this has the additional benefit that it is likely to flush out of the urethra any microbes that may have entered during intercourse. Urinating will have the same effect in women, but they have the disadvantage that sexually transmitted diseases usually develop in the vagina and in the neck of the womb rather than in the urethra.

Women often debate the value and advisability of douching, either to prevent or to treat discharges. Douching is a misguided practice. There is nothing positive in its favor and there is a risk that any infected material could be flushed upward into the uterus rather than be washed out, which is undesirable. The most useful thing that women can do is to soak in a hot bath, allowing the water to flow freely into the vagina. Unless someone is advised to do so by a doctor,

antiseptic lotions or ointments should never be applied either inside or outside the genitals, and strong antiseptic should never be used in the urethra or vagina; it could lead to serious, permanent internal damage.

Where to go for help

If someone thinks that there is even a remote chance that he or she might have some form of STD, the best procedure is to go to a doctor or treatment center immediately to find out. Some hospitals have a separate department of genitourinary medicine where tests can be carried out and advice can be given. Alternatively, anyone worried could telephone the STD National Hotline: 800-227-8922. The AIDS National Hotline is 800-342-2437.

Any information that is obtained at the treatment center is strictly confidential, and patients will usually be referred to by a number so that their anonymity is completely preserved. No information will be given about a patient in response to queries from a spouse or partner, friends, parents, school, employer, or anybody else. Patients' notes are kept separately from any medical records that may exist elsewhere so that there is no possibility of any cross-reference being made between them. The staffs who work at such centers are there to help, not to judge, and the atmosphere is usually very friendly and helpful.

See also: AIDS; Gonorrhea; Herpes; Laboratory tests; Pelvic inflammatory disease; Syphilis

Shiatsu

Originating in Japan, shiatsu is a form of massage that focuses on pressure points lying on the meridians, believed by practitioners to be lines of energy flow in the body. It is claimed to have both physical and psychological benefits.

The movement of any individual practitioner is often called his or her "form." A concern for form is an integral part of shiatsu. The more effort that goes into concentrating on sitting and breathing, the less the mind tries to work out the purpose of it all. When the mind is relaxed, peace of mind can come easily (see Relaxation).

Pressure techniques

There are certain principles that apply to the practice of shiatsu and the techniques of applying the pressure. These are: vertical pressure, which places pressure perpendicular to the surface being worked on; steady pressure, which is sustained and flowing; supporting pressure, which allows the practitioner to rest his or her weight comfortably on the patient without effort or strain; and, finally, equal pressure, a pressure that maintains a uniform weight distribution, causing the patient to be totally relaxed and unaware of the process.

Shiatsu is more vigorous than other forms of massage. Specific areas of the body called meridians, or acupoints, are manipulated (see Acupuncture). The meridians are areas of concentrated energy. The practitioner will sometimes use his or her thumbs, fingers, and even elbows, knees, or feet to apply pressure or to stretch the meridians (see Manipulation).

Visiting a practitioner

Shiatsu is nearly always given at floor level, usually on a padded surface such as a Japanese-style futon. The practitioner must be able to move around the patient's body with ease and agility. If necessary a small and firm pillow should be used.

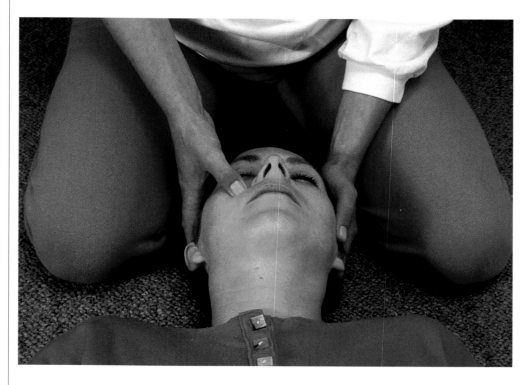

▲ *Shiatsu is a technique that can be applied to all areas of the body. The woman above is receiving a shiatsu facial massage.*

Claimed benefits of shiatsu
Aids digestion
Reduces stress
Improves psychological state
Improves sexual functioning
Aids muscular and skeletal aches
Corrects long-term posture problems
Improves general sense of well-being

Both the practitioner and the client should wear loose, comfortable clothing. For giving shiatsu to the feet, hands, face, and neck, a thin cotton fiber cloth is often used. The thin layer of cotton between the practitioner and the patient allows the former to move easily from one position to the next without stretching or pinching the skin.

The room in which the massage is taking place should be warm, dimly lit, and quiet. These conditions produce the perfect state for both the body and the mind to be in a complete state of relaxation. This allows the patient to receive the maximum benefit from the treatment.

Shiatsu can be practiced at any time of the day. However, the ideal time is unique to each client. At the end of the day it can be a good time for relaxation, but it can also be an invigorating start to each day.

Since a shiatsu session can make a client sleepy and even euphoric, it is a good idea for him or her to remain calm for about 15 minutes after the treatment to let the mind

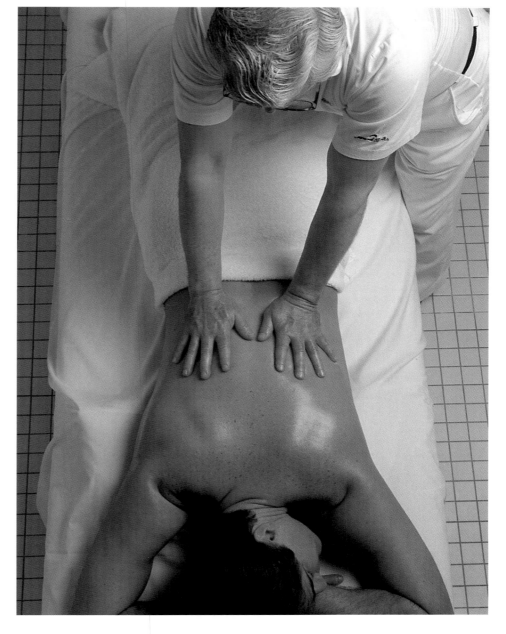

▲ *During shiatsu treatment, the patient lies on a padded surface near the floor. The room is dimly lit, warm, and quiet so that the patient can feel totally relaxed.*

resurface slowly and the body to wake itself up. A session usually lasts for about an hour—no longer, since this can be detrimental to the benefits of the treatment. Sometimes a 30-minute session is enough. A client can have up to three sessions a week, although most people have only one. If the client is being treated for a specific problem, such as a sore shoulder or painful hip, he or she may require a series of treatments that can be carried out over several weeks.

Benefits

The main aim of a shiatsu practitioner is to work out the strengths and weaknesses in the patient and to assess his or her ability to respond to treatment, to stimulate energy sources, and to restore harmony to the body's systems. The prompting of the meridians and the points breaks up blocked energy and draws it toward the weaker areas.

Shiatsu is based on the Chinese theory of the yin and the yang (see Chinese Medicine). According to the theory, an extreme of one can transform to its opposite. In a situation where there is tension and pain, the firmer pressure disperses the blockage and the yang becomes yin, releasing the tension and creating relaxation (see Tension). On the other hand, in weak areas a softer, lingering pressure can draw energy to the areas, turning the yin to yang and reenergizing the body.

Shiatsu treatment is a direct interaction between the practitioner and the patient, and the success of the treatment may depend on the level of commitment the patient shows his or her practitioner.

See also: Acupressure; Massage; Mind-body therapy

Shingles

Questions and Answers

My grandmother had shingles, and the rash seemed to encircle half her body like a belt. Is this usual?

Yes. The main characteristic of the disease is that it is an infection that nearly always spreads out from the spinal cord through the nerves of sensation. Each nerve supplies an area of skin called a dermatome. These are arranged down the surface of the body like a series of belts or horizontal stripes. Normally, shingles will affect one nerve's dermatome on only one side of the body, although more than one nerve can be affected.

When my father had shingles it was so painful that he couldn't move for a week. Is this normal?

Yes, it is normal for the condition to be painful in the early stages, but the pain will often diminish as soon as the rash has broken out. Usually the surface tenderness is not too bad after the rash has settled down, but often the pain, called postherpetic neuralgia, will persist over the affected area.

Is it true that if you have shingles down both sides, you will die if the two areas meet up?

No; this is an old wives' tale. No one dies of shingles, although the disease can occur in people who are ill with other diseases and may compound their deterioration.

Are elderly people at risk of catching shingles from children who have chicken pox?

No. Although both diseases are caught from the same virus, there is very little evidence that shingles can be caught from people with chicken pox. However, it is possible for infection to work the other way around; people can get chicken pox from someone who suffers from shingles.

This painful disease is caused by the same virus as chicken pox and affects mainly adults. It can be very debilitating but will not usually cause long-term damage, and complete recovery nearly always occurs.

Shingles is a very painful but not dangerous disease that tends to affect the elderly and the sick. The medical name for the condition is herpes zoster, which is Greek for "creeping girdle," referring to the way in which the disease shows up as a beltlike rash around the body.

Causes

Shingles and chicken pox are both caused by the same virus, although the two diseases are quite different (see Viruses). The only similarity is that they both produce a rash with vesicles (fluid-filled clear spots) on the skin (see Skin and Skin Diseases).

Chicken pox and shingles tend to occur in very different age groups. Chicken pox primarily affects children, whereas shingles is very rare in childhood; most cases crop up after the age of 40. After an attack of chicken pox, the viruses travel up the sensory nerves to the nerve ganglia near the spinal cord. They remain dormant there for years, kept in check by the immune system. Shingles occurs when the level of this immune surveillance drops (see Chicken Pox).

Symptoms

Shingles starts with pain felt on the surface of the skin where the disease is going to strike. This pain may get worse over the next few days, and the skin will redden. At this point the rash starts to break out, with little vesicles forming on the skin. The pain tends to diminish as the rash advances but it may still be severe. The rash will often creep around one side of the body, causing the characteristic beltlike condition. The areas most commonly affected are the chest and upper part of the abdomen; the lower abdomen, limbs, neck, and face are involved less often.

The disease has this beltlike appearance because the virus spreads down sensory nerves from the spinal cord. These nerves emerge in pairs from between each of the vertebrae in the backbone, and each one supplies a band of skin called a dermatome on one half of the body (see Spinal Cord).

Once the rash has appeared, it will persist for several days and the vesicles may even run together to form a mat of affected skin with a crust over it. Eventually, though, the rash will clear, leaving normal skin behind. Sometimes there will be some depigmentation or minor scarring. The pain associated with shingles usually disappears with the rash or soon after.

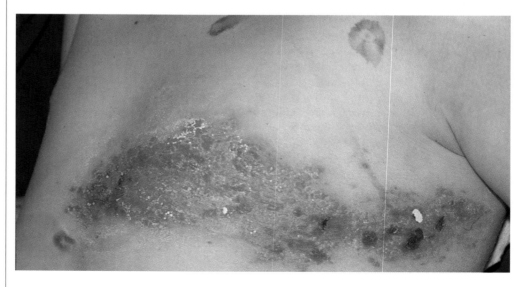

▲ *The shingles rash, caused by a virus, creeps around the body, forming a kind of band.*

Aside from affecting mainly older people, shingles is also found typically in patients suffering from other diseases that tend to suppress the activity of the immune system, such as leukemia or a lymphoma (see Immune System; Leukemia; Lymphoma).

Unusual forms of the disease

There may be variations in the disease. It is thought that shingles can actually occur without the telltale rash. This is very difficult to prove, but it is a likely explanation for the occasional patient who has severe pain in the area where one would expect a patch of shingles to develop.

Sometimes the disease is not confined to the sensory part of the nervous system, and muscle weakness may occur with an attack of shingles (see Muscles). This suggests that the motor nerves as well as the nerves of sensation are involved.

Shingles can also affect areas supplied by the nerves of the head that arise not from the spinal cord but from the brain. Although any area of the face can be involved, it usually affects the ophthalmic branch of the trigeminal nerve, the main nerve of sensation in the face. Generally the skin around the eye is affected but sometimes the eye itself is involved (see Eyes and Eyesight). Another area that may be affected is the ear; in this case the condition is called Ramsay Hunt's syndrome (after the neurologist who first described it).

Dangers

The main danger of the disease is the development of postherpetic neuralgia: that

▼ *This electron micrograph shows one particle of the shingles virus, herpes zoster (center), magnified 200,000 times.*

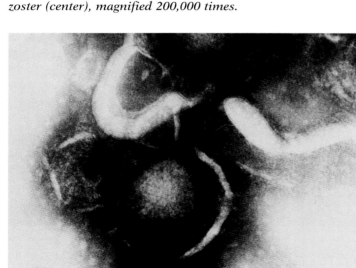

DISTRIBUTION OF DERMATOMES

The area of skin supplied by one spinal nerve is called a dermatome. Dermatomes extend around the body from front to back, never crossing the midline. The different colors represent dermatomes associated with different segments of the spinal cord. Shingles spreads along the dermatomes, hence its characteristic appearance.

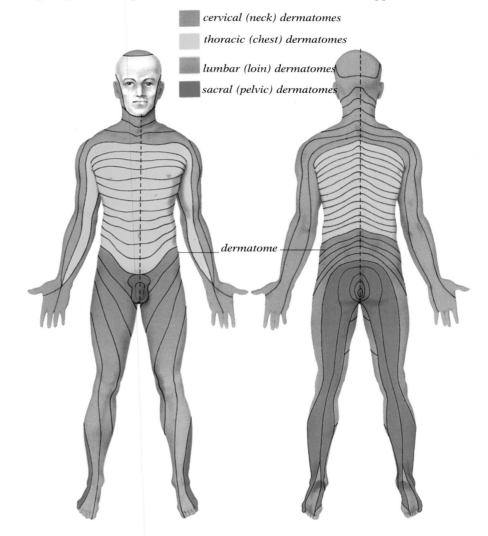

- *cervical (neck) dermatomes*
- *thoracic (chest) dermatomes*
- *lumbar (loin) dermatomes*
- *sacral (pelvic) dermatomes*

dermatome

is, the pain associated with the condition does not abate as the rash disappears. This is more likely to happen when the trigeminal nerve of the face is involved. This form of the disease may also be dangerous, since the eye may become involved, leading to inflammation and, in rare cases, even blindness.

Treatment

The antiviral drug aciclovir, sold under the trade name of Zovirax, has valuable specific action against the herpes zoster virus. Although it cannot entirely cure the disease, it will markedly lessen the severity of the symptoms and reduce the probability or duration of postherpetic neuralgia. To be most effective, however, Zovirax—which is taken by mouth—must be started as early as possible, ideally at the first indication of shingles. Delay in starting to take the drug is never justified.

See also: **Herpes; Nervous system; Rashes**

Shivering

Questions and Answers

When it is cold I shiver long before others do. Why?

This is probably because your thermostat is set differently from theirs. Everyone has internal mechanisms that govern vital processes such as thirst, appetite, sleep, or temperature, and each person's setting is different. You may find your setting inconvenient, but you are not at any risk.

When my little girl had measles she shivered so violently that the whole bed shook. Why did this happen?

In many feverish illnesses germs or toxins push the "normal" setting of the brain thermostat to a higher level. The body immediately reacts as if it were too cold, and produces more heat. Its most efficient way of doing this is rapidly repeated muscle contractions—shivering.

How do you tell the difference between severe shivering and an epileptic attack?

If the shivering is only slight or the epileptic attack is severe, with the patient falling to the ground, jerking violently, and losing consciousness, there is little doubt. But if the shivering is severe or the epileptic attack mild, it may not be easy to distinguish the two just on appearance. If the circumstances are inappropriate for shivering—for example, if the attack occurs on a hot summer's day—then epilepsy is more likely. If there is any doubt, consult your doctor, who will arrange for neurologic tests.

Is shivering usually a sign of illness?

Shivering in cold weather is normal and one of the ways in which the body warms up. At other times it is a sign that something has upset the body's temperature control system, and is usually associated with a sharp rise in temperature.

Everyone knows what it's like to shiver in cold weather; this involuntary shaking movement of the skin muscles is one mechanism with which the body tries to keep warm by raising its temperature.

Because shivering is a familiar sensation and one that people tend to take for granted, they rarely stop to think about either the mechanisms involved or its purpose. Normal shivering consists of uncontrollable shaking that usually involves the whole body. It is uncontrollable in the sense that it cannot be stopped or started voluntarily by an act of will. There are several other body reactions that are similar, and shivering needs to be distinguished from them.

A response to cold

The most important feature of shivering is that it is a response to cold and that its purpose is to warm up the body. Trembling, on the other hand, is also an involuntary action that involves generalized shaking; however, the stimulus is not cold but fear, shock, or an emotional disorder such as hysteria (see Hysteria).

Shaking or trembling that affects a particular part of the body is characteristic of some disorders of the brain or nerves—for example, Parkinson's disease or alcoholism. In medical parlance this is called tremor (see Alcoholism; Parkinson's Disease; Tremor).

Shaking that is more severe or dramatic than is usually associated with shivering is called a convulsion or fit. This is characteristic of epilepsy and can usually be distinguished from true shivering (see Epilepsy). However, in slight attacks the distinction between the two may not be very great. The fact that the surrounding temperature is not low enough to account for shivering may be an indication that the shaking is really a minor convulsion and not the body's reaction to cold.

Temperature control

Shivering is an important mechanism in the body's complex and vital temperature control system. The temperature of the human body is normally in the region of 97°F to 99°F (36°C to 37°C) and

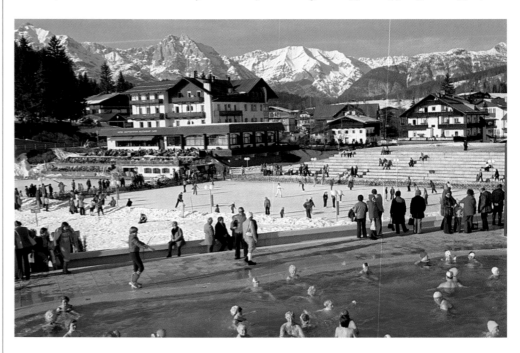

▲ *The best of both worlds: people having fun in a heated outdoor swimming pool in a spectacular setting. Swimming keeps them warm; the shivering starts later.*

remains remarkably constant, no matter how hot or cold the weather may be. This is not an accident, but a necessity, since this is the temperature at which the body's metabolism, the intricate complex of interrelated chemical reactions, functions best (see Metabolism).

In fact, some of these metabolic reactions are so sensitive to temperature that if there are substantial departures from the normal temperature range for very long, they will be severely affected. Unless the situation is rectified and a return to normal body temperature is achieved, a progressive breakdown in the usual metabolic processes will occur until a point is reached at which life can no longer continue. This is what happens when people have very high temperatures, called hyperpyrexia, or, perhaps in circumstances of exposure, very low temperatures resulting in the condition called hypothermia.

Thus mechanisms for keeping the body's internal temperature at the right level, irrespective of how hot or cold the outside temperature is, are vital for our survival. These mechanisms, of which shivering is one of the most important, are under the control of the hypothalamus, one of the nonthinking, automatic centers in the brain (see Hypothalamus). These kinds of temperature-regulating mechanisms are most efficient in healthy adults; they are much less effective in infants and elderly people, whose susceptibility to serious effects from temperature changes is therefore much greater. This is shown by the high incidence of hypothermia among elderly people.

The right temperature

The mechanisms by which our bodies maintain the correct temperature are ingenious. If the temperature-sensitive nerve endings, which are situated throughout the body (see Nervous System), inform the thermostat in the hypothalamus that the temperature is becoming too high, a well-ordered chain of events takes place. Messages are sent to the arteries in the deeper parts of the body, and these become narrower so that less blood flows through them. At the same time, the blood vessels just below the surface of the skin are allowed to open wider; the result is that a higher proportion of the body's blood is flowing close to the surface of the skin. Here it can be cooled by the air and excess heat can be radiated away. If the body cannot be cooled sufficiently by radiation, the sweating

HOW SHIVERING OCCURS

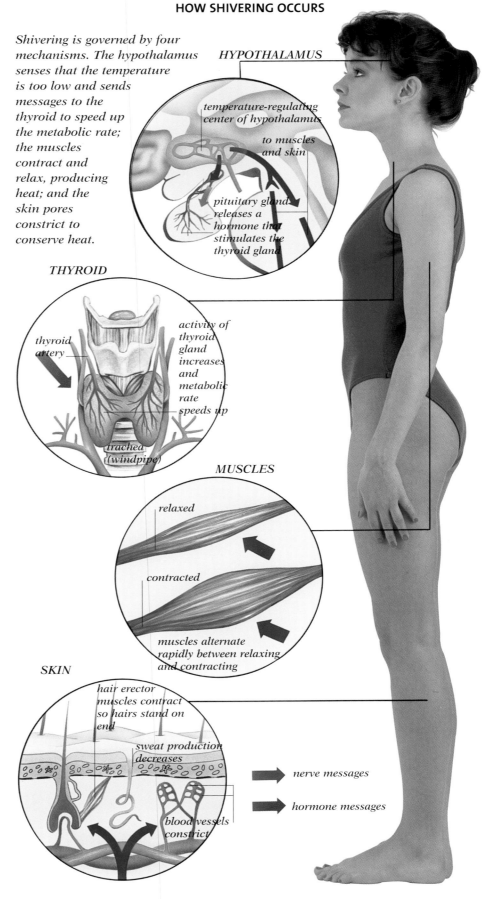

Shivering is governed by four mechanisms. The hypothalamus senses that the temperature is too low and sends messages to the thyroid to speed up the metabolic rate; the muscles contract and relax, producing heat; and the skin pores constrict to conserve heat.

HYPOTHALAMUS

temperature-regulating center of hypothalamus

to muscles and skin

pituitary gland releases a hormone that stimulates the thyroid gland

THYROID

thyroid artery

activity of thyroid gland increases and metabolic rate speeds up

trachea (windpipe)

MUSCLES

relaxed

contracted

muscles alternate rapidly between relaxing and contracting

SKIN

hair erector muscles contract so hairs stand on end

sweat production decreases

blood vessels constrict

→ nerve messages

→ hormone messages

mechanism comes into operation. Sweat is secreted onto the skin, and, as it evaporates, it cools both the skin and the blood flowing just beneath it, bringing the temperature down (see Perspiration).

If, on the other hand, the outside temperature drops sufficiently for the body to react, then different mechanisms are brought into play to conserve or boost the body's internal temperature. The first of these, once again controlled by the hypothalamus, is a sequence to change the pattern of the blood circulation. Blood is directed away from the surface of the skin to the deeper regions of the body, so that heat loss through radiation is cut to a minimum. When, however, it is so cold that this mechanism is not enough, the additional and closely related measures of so-called goose pimples, a sudden puckering of the skin, and shivering come into play to try to increase the body's heat.

Goose pimples and shivering

The effectiveness of these reactions is based on the fact that the body's natural heat is produced as a side effect of metabolizing or burning up food materials. This happens to people most extensively when energy needs to be produced for muscular activity, such as after a long run. Thus any muscular activity will produce more heat and raise the temperature of the body; and this is what goose pimples and shivering achieve. The puckering of the skin that takes place when goose pimples are formed is the result of contraction of the muscle fibers in the skin. In a sense it is an involuntary isometric exercise (see Isometrics). Shivering is much more energetic, and therefore a much more effective, heat-producing activity. It involves rapid alternating contraction and relaxation of the muscles of the skin.

Abnormal shivering

Shivering is normally a response to low external temperatures. When it occurs at other times it is said to be abnormal. A common example of this type of shivering is the bout of violent shaking that people sometimes experience as the body tries to raise its temperature rapidly. This happens with certain feverish illnesses, such as influenza, pneumonia, and tonsillitis; this type of shivering is called a rigor.

The explanation is that, in the course of the illness, the body suddenly produces an unusually large quantity of heat. This happens because the disease germs reset the thermostat in the hypothalamus to a higher level. The body systems read this as an indication that it is too cold and that heat is urgently required. The result is shivering, which, if the thermostat is set very high, may be violent. Later, however, the body's heat-losing mechanisms redress the balance by means of heavy sweating, another symptom of feverish illness.

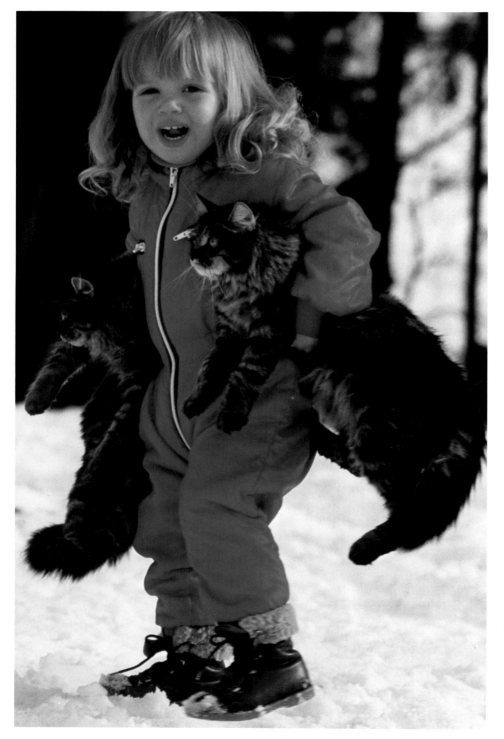

◄ *If you insulate yourself from the cold, you won't shiver: the differences between internal and external temperatures will be stabilized. This little girl is warmly bundled up; her cats have built-in insulation thanks to their thick fur.*

See also: **Fevers; Hypothermia; Influenza; Temperature**

Shock

Questions and Answers

If you suffer from shock after a serious accident, do you have to be treated in an intensive care unit?

If your injuries are so severe that you have gone into shock through loss of blood, you might need to have intensive care to see you over the immediate danger. However, if your blood loss is fairly easy to control in the emergency room, and you recover well after having had a blood transfusion, then you should be well enough to be looked after on a general floor.

After prostate surgery my father went into shock. Did the surgeon make a mistake, or was there some other cause for this condition?

Your father probably had what is called septic shock, in which a bacterium finds its way into the blood during surgery and causes an infection. There is little that the surgeon can do to guard against this; it is a known risk of surgical interference with the urinary system. However, if the shock is noticed early it should respond to treatment with antibiotics.

My boyfriend recently fell off his motorbike. Two days later he began to have severe shortness of breath, something the doctors called shock lung. What is this?

Shock, or wet, lung is more properly called adult respiratory distress syndrome (ARDS). It is a disorder of the lungs associated with some forms of severe trauma that do not involve the chest. Its exact causes, however, are poorly understood. What seems to happen is that damaged tissue releases something that makes the blood vessels in the lungs leak so that the lungs fill up with fluid. When shock lung occurs, the patient is placed on a respirator. This supplies properly oxygenated blood to the body until the lungs recover their normal function.

A person who is pale, cold, and clammy after an accident is almost certainly suffering from shock. Speedy treatment by blood transfusion can often be a lifesaver to the shock victim.

There is a big difference between the way that most people use the word "shock" and the way that doctors use it. In an everyday sense, people talk about a sudden event giving rise to an unpleasant surprise, or shock. On the other hand, to the doctor, "shock" is a medical condition in which the failure of the circulatory system, for one reason or another, is a central feature (see Circulatory System). Sometimes the different uses of the word cause confusion.

Psychological shocks

It would be wrong to ignore totally the effects of sudden unpleasant psychological shocks: they can often cause considerable distress and can even precipitate serious psychological illness. However, this is likely only in people already at risk of some sort of psychological illness (see Psychology).

Sudden psychological shocks can cause collapse on their own: people may faint at the sight of a gruesome automobile accident, and it is not uncommon for people to faint when they are given bad news. Also, an unpleasant or horrifying experience can lead to the development of serious symptoms of anxiety that may last for some time: this is particularly likely in the case of victims of violent crime (see Anxiety).

One of the psychological shocks that most people have to experience at some time is the death of a close friend or relative. If the death occurs unexpectedly, the initial horror of the event may leave someone numbed, and the deep sadness may take some time to sink in. Even if the death is expected, the finality of bereavement is still an event that will change a person's life and outlook (see Death; Grief).

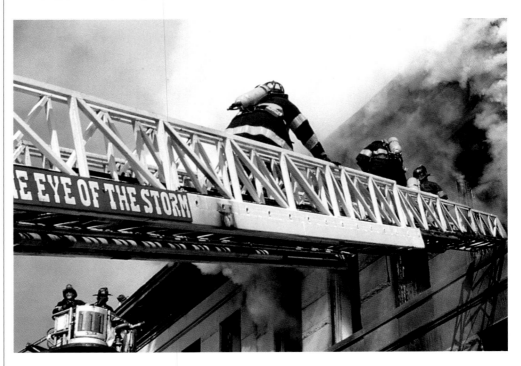

▲ *In second- or third-degree burns affecting more than 10 percent of the body surface, the victim will usually be in a state of shock. This condition is provoked by the loss of large quantities of fluid (and its constituent proteins) from the burned area. Shock can be fatal if not rapidly treated by intravenous fluid replacement.*

Questions and Answers

Just after the death of his wife, my friend of mine seemed quite calm, but a few weeks later he became really miserable. Was he suffering from delayed shock?

People often talk about "delayed shock," though to the doctor this term does not have any special meaning. It is most often used to describe the way in which the full sadness of bereavement may take days or even weeks to sink in. The period immediately after loss can seem unreal, and the bereaved person can be in a daze.

My father died after going into shock after a heart attack. Could he have been saved by surgery?

No, it is very unlikely. The sort of shock that happens after a heart attack is called cardiogenic shock, and the problem is caused because the damaged heart lacks the strength to pump adequate blood around the body. It is very hard to treat because the only way to get the blood around the body is by making the already damaged heart work harder.

My best friend was killed in an automobile crash, and I felt weak and wobbly for days. Was I suffering from shock?

The shock of losing your best friend was undoubtedly responsible for the unusual symptoms you experienced. However, doctors are much more likely to use the word "shock" to describe the sort of collapse that follows from the loss of blood after an accident, rather than the psychological shock that you experienced.

Can a person die of shock?

If you are talking about the medical use of the word (meaning collapse of the heart and circulation), then certainly a shock can be fatal. However, psychological shock alone is unlikely to cause death in a fit person, although it might be fatal in someone already suffering from a heart condition.

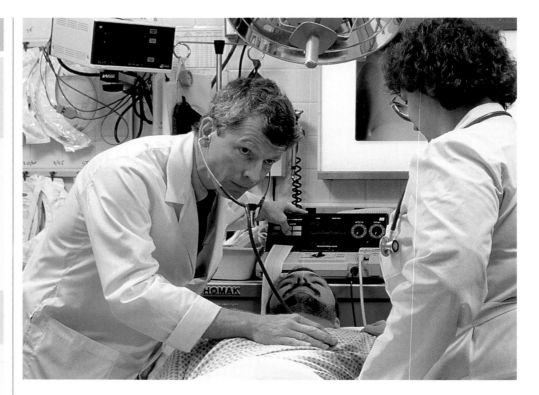

▲ *A male patient receives emergency coronary care from a hospital trauma team. A heart attack is one of the most common causes of shock. Careful and constant monitoring of the patient's heart rate is required to help restore stability.*

These different shocks are the bumps and bruises that people usually have to experience during their lives. If the shocks are severe enough and a person is vulnerable, then they may take their toll and leave some psychological scar. However, these events are not what shock means in the medical sense; it is something much more immediate and easy to recognize. The failure of the circulation is the basic problem, and treatment is the province of the hospital physician or surgeon rather than the counselor or psychiatrist (see Counseling; Psychiatry).

What is shock?

Shock develops because of the way the heart and circulation work together. If for some reason the heart fails to pump properly or there is not enough blood for it to pump, then insufficient blood will be circulating to sustain the vital functions. This can be brought on by a variety of factors, ranging from loss of large amounts of blood to failure of the heart itself (see Blood; Heart).

For the heart to pump in the correct manner, it has to be primed with blood, and there must be some blood in the system for the heart to get up enough pressure to push the blood around. Normally, blood leaves the heart and travels throughout the body in arteries. Larger arteries give way to smaller ones, called arterioles, which have thick muscular walls (see Arteries and Artery Disease). If blood pressure goes down, these arterioles can constrict so that there is less space for the blood to flow through. This causes the pressure to rise again because the blood is being squeezed into a smaller space than before.

This system of constriction of the arterioles, called vasoconstriction, is one of the body's ways of maintaining the correct blood pressure when things go wrong. If the pressure falls too low, blood cannot flow around all the tissues. In fact, when the system fails—after excessive bleeding, for example—shock occurs.

Hypovolemic shock

There are several types of shock. One of the most common results from the massive loss of fluid (blood or water) that can follow from critical injury or illness. This is termed "hypovolemic shock." Second- and third-degree burns can provoke shock because of the extensive fluid loss that occurs in the burned area.

MEASURING CENTRAL VENOUS PRESSURE

Accurate monitoring of the blood pressure in the right atrium of the heart can be vital in cases of shock. The subclavian vein is found with a syringe (1) and a catheter introduced into the atrium (2). The blood pressure is measured with a manometer (3).

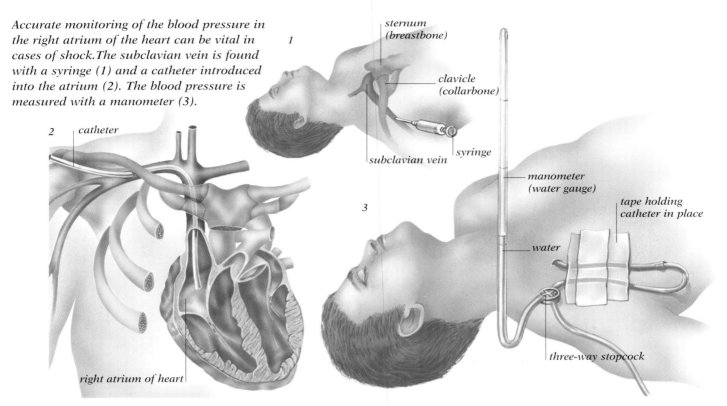

Fluid loss does not result only from accidents. It is not uncommon for there to be serious bleeding from ulcers in the stomach (see Ulcers). In these cases, large amounts of blood are either vomited or passed through the rectum. Patients suffering from this sort of gastrointestinal bleeding can arrive in the emergency room in a state of extreme shock.

Large blood loss can also occur during childbirth (intrapartum hemorrhage), though with blood transfusions shock under these circumstances has become increasingly rare. Similarly, diarrhea, particularly in young children, can cause severe dehydration, which in turn can provoke shock (see Diarrhea).

Septic shock

Some infections can cause shock, though in this case the mechanism underlying the shock is different. Infection in the blood may lead to the production of toxins (see Infection and Infectious Diseases). These toxins seem to have a direct effect on the blood vessels in the tissues, causing the venules (very small veins) to become widened and very leaky. Blood becomes pooled in the venules, and insufficient amounts return to the heart and therefore the blood pressure falls. This is known as endotoxic or septic shock.

Cardiogenic shock

Another major cause of shock results from disease of the heart itself. This is called cardiogenic shock, and its main cause is an extensive heart attack. The heart muscle is partly destroyed by the heart attack, and the more that is destroyed the more severe the effects of the attack will be. When more than 30 percent has been destroyed, shock is likely to develop because the remaining heart muscle simply lacks the power to pump enough blood (see Heart Attack; Heart Disease).

Neurogenic shock

This occurs when the brain is starved of oxygen, causing a collapse of the nervous system and a complete loss of control over the circulation (see Nervous System).

Anaphylactic shock

Another type of shock is a very rare and sometimes fatal allergic reaction. Common allergens that can cause such extreme reactions include insect stings, drugs, and some common foods such as nuts (see Allergies).

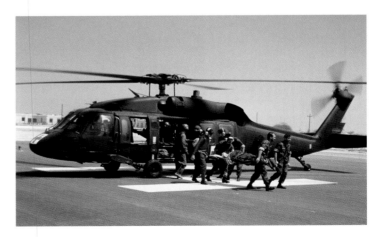

▲ *Early skilled assistance, in this case the replacement of lost body fluids with clear plasma, can be lifesaving to the shock victim. Many lives can now be saved on the battlefield by early treatment and rapid transport to a base hospital.*

Symptoms of shock

People with shock tend to have a similar appearance. They are pale and often cold and clammy to the touch; when the blood pressure is measured, it is found to be critically low. One exception to this, however, is during septic shock, where, despite the low blood pressure, the patient is warm to the touch.

The pallor is caused by lack of blood in the skin: blood has been forced from the skin by the vasoconstriction. The coldness is because the blood, which carries body heat, is sent back into the body's core.

It might seem strange that people are sweaty and cold at the same time, but the autonomic nervous system, which is responsible for running the body's unconscious functions, not only causes the vasoconstriction but also causes the adrenal glands to release epinephrine, which in turn makes the sweat glands work.

Effects of shock

As well as the immediate, dangerous effects of shock, it can create other, long-term problems. The two most important of these affect the kidneys and the lungs. When shock develops and there is insufficient blood passing through the kidneys, acute renal failure can develop. The kidneys stop passing urine, and waste products, particularly urea (a breakdown product of protein), start to build up in the blood. If the shock is dealt with fairly quickly, the kidneys are likely to recover speedily. However, the process can be slow and dialysis may be required for days or even weeks (see Kidney Dialysis).

If shock has stopped the kidneys from working, the situation may deteriorate even further. The blood supply to the brain may become inadequate, and, as a consequence, confusion and then unconsciousness may set in. The skin can sometimes progress from being cold and clammy to a gangrenous condition resulting from the poor blood flow (see Gangrene). When it has gone this far, there is very little hope for the patient.

The effect of shock on the lungs is a comparatively newly recognized condition. The effect, called shock lung, can occur even in apparently fit young people who have had large-volume blood transfusions after an accident. Patients who have this complication become breathless, and the level of oxygen in the blood starts to fall. There is also extensive shadowing on chest X rays.

What happens is this: the lung acts as a filter to any abnormal substances circulating in the blood, and, because it is common for transfused blood to contain a few little clumps of cells, these get caught up in the fine capillaries in the lungs and cause a blockage. The basis of most treatment is to take over the function of the lungs by placing the patient on a respirator.

Treatment of shock

The aim of treatment for shock in all its forms is to try to return the volume of blood in the circulation to normal so that the heart can pump normally and an adequate amount of blood flows to the tissues. When blood loss has been the cause of shock, then the

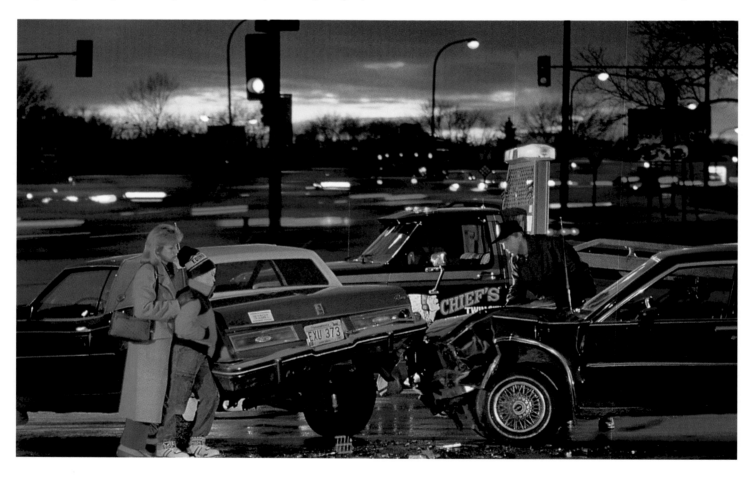

▲ *Car accidents are a major cause of injury and shock. Patients suffering from shock need constant attention, as their condition can change dramatically at any moment. They should be kept cool to conserve blood vital for the heart and brain.*

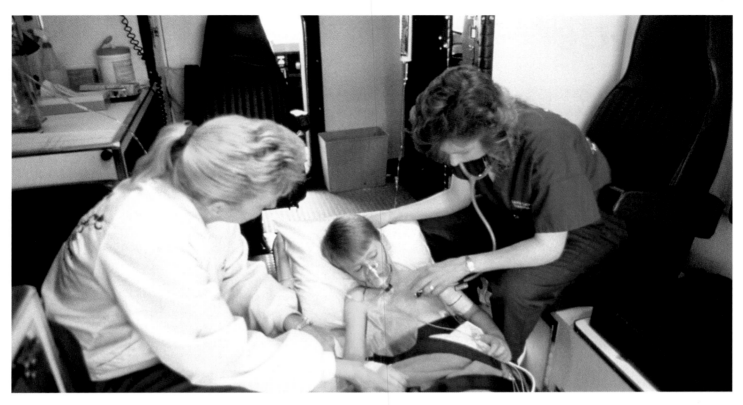

▲ *Paramedics care for an injured child in a large ambulance van immediately after a traffic accident.*

treatment is simply a transfusion of the correct amount of blood to bring the volume back to normal. When the shock is due to septicemia, the body still needs fluid even though the blood is pooled in the blood vessels. In this instance, clear fluids in the form of salt or sugar solutions or protein fluids such as plasma are used (see Plasma).

However, there can be problems in giving large amounts of blood or fluid to older patients, since these additional fluids can overload the heart and lead to heart failure. Doctors have to get around this problem, and to do this they have to keep a balance between having too much and too little fluid in the circulation. They measure fluid by checking the pressure in the right atrium of the heart.

This pressure measurement is called the central venous pressure (CVP). To take the pressure, a fine tube is passed into a vein in the leg or neck and the pressure is measured outside the body using a simple column of water. If the pressure is too high there is too much fluid; if it is too low there is not enough.

Shock caused by a heart attack (cardiogenic shock) cannot, however, be treated by a blood transfusion. Common forms of treatment include drugs that make the heart work harder (inotropic drugs such as digoxin) and drugs that reduce the amount of work it has to do. Drugs that make it work harder, however, can place a great strain on a weakened heart.

One technique that gets around some of these problems is a device called a balloon pump. A long sausage-shaped balloon is inserted at the top of the aorta, the biggest artery from the heart, and connected by a tube to a pump outside the body. The balloon is inflated between heartbeats to help force blood out along the arteries, reducing the amount of work the heart has to do and raising the blood pressure. When the balloon deflates, it allows more blood to be pumped from the heart into the aorta; when it inflates, it forces the blood around.

First aid for shock

In giving first aid for shock, it is important to diagnose and treat the cause of shock, rather than to diagnose and treat the shock itself. Very often the cause of shock is obvious: in a traffic accident, for example, the cause is generally major blood loss. The victim will often be dizzy; he or she may vomit or completely lose consciousness. The skin color will be very pale and the pulse rapid.

The victim should be laid flat with his or her legs slightly raised; this stimulates blood flow to the brain. He or she should be kept cool to ensure that blood continues to circulate to the heart and brain. Giving him or her liquids should be avoided, as these may make surgery difficult once the patient has reached the hospital. Above all, it is important to make sure that an ambulance is called promptly.

Outlook

The outlook for the patient with shock depends a lot on the fitness of the person before the condition developed and on what was the cause of the shock.

A fit person who loses a lot of blood in a traffic accident but whose injuries are not too serious should do well after a blood transfusion and treatment for the physical damage. However, an older patient who gets shock caused by infection after surgery is at much greater risk. Also, someone who develops kidney failure or shock lung is in a much more risky situation. The outlook for the person with cardiogenic shock is at present very poor.

> *See also:* **Bites and stings; Blood pressure; Blood transfusion; Burns; Emergencies; Fainting; Hemorrhage; Sepsis; Unconsciousness**

Shoulder

Questions and Answers

My teenage son tends to walk and sit badly, with his shoulders rounded. Is there a medical reason why he should be encouraged to improve his posture?

Yes. Sitting and walking with round shoulders may give rise to permanent deformity and is often associated with pain and disability of the arms and hands. Your son's round-shouldered stance may reflect an excessive degree of self-consciousness, a common problem of adolescence. Instead of being tempted to nag him to sit and walk in a more upright way, which will help only temporarily and is likely to do more harm than good, try to give your son a psychological boost so that he will have good reason to hold his head up.

Why is it that after a good night's sleep I often wake up with a pain in my shoulder?

When you sleep soundly and don't move about much in bed, certain muscles, depending on the exact position in which you are lying, tend to stiffen up and the nerves in that area may be subjected to abnormal pressure. For both reasons, pain can result. Try to do some loosening-up exercises in the morning, but if the pain persists throughout the day it would be wise to consult your doctor. If you tend to go to sleep in one position, try a change. You may find this is the ideal solution.

Is it true that gastric trouble can cause a pain in the shoulder?

Yes. Because of the way in which the body's nerves are arranged, a variety of disorders of the chest and abdomen—such as angina, lung disease, stomach ulcers, and diseases of the liver, gallbladder, and pancreas—can cause pain in the shoulders and arms. You should therefore tell your doctor about any such pains.

The shoulders are the joints that connect the arms to the body and allow a vast range of arm and shoulder movements. However, the exceptional mobility of the shoulders makes them prone to a number of specific complaints.

The joint at the shoulder is the link between the upper arm bone, called the humerus, and the triangular-shaped scapula, or shoulder blade (see Bones). Anatomically, the joint is classified as the ball-and-socket type because a ball-shaped projection at the top of the humerus articulates with a socket in the scapula. This socket, called the glenoid cavity or fossa, is actually rather shallow so that the head of the humerus perches on the cup, like a golf ball on a tee, rather than slotting deep into it. This allows the arm to rotate through a complete circle in several different planes.

The movement of the bones at the shoulder is assisted by lubricated synovial membranes between the surfaces of the two bones (see Membranes). Unlike other joints, the ligaments that are intended to hold the bone in place are not particularly strong; that is why dislocation of the shoulder is common (see Ligaments). Much stability is provided by muscles that also control movement. The most important of these muscles are the series of fan-shaped ones that run from the scapula to the top of the humerus and to the end of the collarbone, or clavicle—the bone that runs from the breastbone, or sternum, to the top of the shoulder joint. These are the deltoid, pectoralis major, and trapezius muscles. The biceps and triceps muscles, located at the front and back of the upper arm, respectively, are also involved in shoulder movements (see Muscles).

Shoulder problems

The shoulder is prone to a number of injuries common to most other joints of the body, but there are one or two problems that are particularly associated with the shoulder.

Dislocation of the shoulder is a common problem with this joint because of its rather loose construction. A heavy fall may be sufficient initially to cause the injury. After a first dislocation, the shoulder often dislocates increasingly easily, even while a person is performing mundane tasks such as housework, digging the garden, or even decorating.

When the shoulder is dislocated, the ball-shaped projection at the end of the humerus can be seen as a bulge in the upper arm. The immediate treatment for a dislocated shoulder is manipulation of the joint to realign the bones correctly. In the long term, however, surgery will be needed to tighten the ligaments and provide a permanent cure.

A broken collarbone is the most common break associated with the shoulder and is an occupational hazard of many sports (see Fractures; Sports Injury). The telltale symptom of a

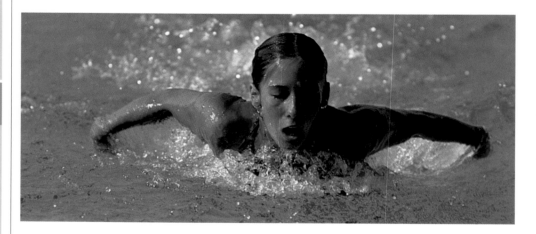

▲ *The butterfly action of this swimmer captures the power and mobility of the shoulder joint. Swimming is an ideal shoulder exercise, because it both builds up muscles and keeps the joint mobile.*

STRUCTURE OF THE SHOULDER

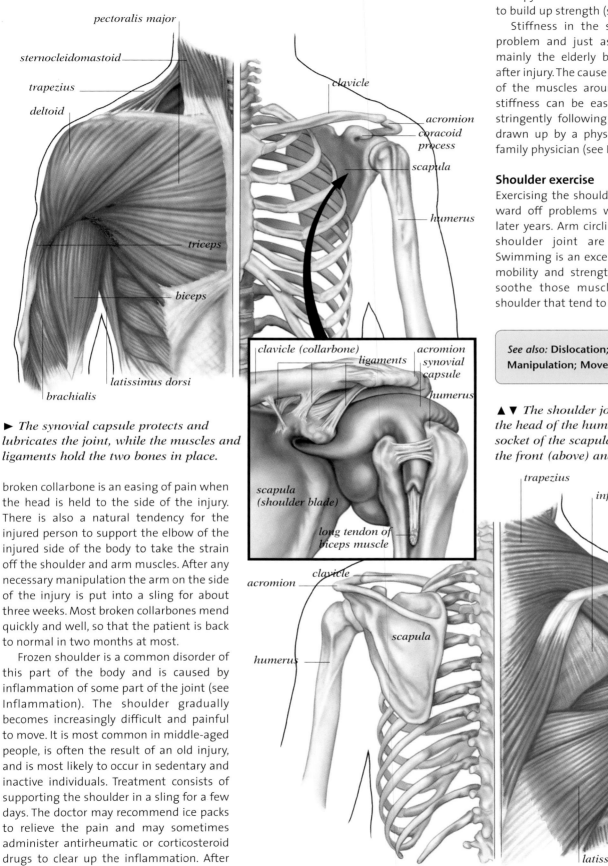

pectoralis major

sternocleidomastoid

trapezius

deltoid

triceps

biceps

latissimus dorsi

brachialis

clavicle

acromion
coracoid
process

scapula

humerus

clavicle (collarbone)

ligaments

acromion
synovial
capsule

humerus

scapula
(shoulder blade)

long tendon of
biceps muscle

acromion

clavicle

humerus

scapula

▶ *The synovial capsule protects and lubricates the joint, while the muscles and ligaments hold the two bones in place.*

broken collarbone is an easing of pain when the head is held to the side of the injury. There is also a natural tendency for the injured person to support the elbow of the injured side of the body to take the strain off the shoulder and arm muscles. After any necessary manipulation the arm on the side of the injury is put into a sling for about three weeks. Most broken collarbones mend quickly and well, so that the patient is back to normal in two months at most.

Frozen shoulder is a common disorder of this part of the body and is caused by inflammation of some part of the joint (see Inflammation). The shoulder gradually becomes increasingly difficult and painful to move. It is most common in middle-aged people, is often the result of an old injury, and is most likely to occur in sedentary and inactive individuals. Treatment consists of supporting the shoulder in a sling for a few days. The doctor may recommend ice packs to relieve the pain and may sometimes administer antirheumatic or corticosteroid drugs to clear up the inflammation. After the inflammation has cleared up, physical

therapy is used both to loosen the joint and to build up strength (see Physical Therapy).

Stiffness in the shoulder is a similar problem and just as common. It affects mainly the elderly but sometimes occurs after injury. The cause is tearing or weakness of the muscles around the joint; but the stiffness can be eased or even cured by stringently following an exercise program drawn up by a physical therapist or your family physician (see Exercise).

Shoulder exercise

Exercising the shoulders regularly can help ward off problems with the shoulders in later years. Arm circling and circling of the shoulder joint are good for mobility. Swimming is an excellent exercise for both mobility and strength, and can also help soothe those muscles in the neck and shoulder that tend to tense up under stress.

See also: Dislocation; Joints; Manipulation; Movement; Stiffness

▲▼ *The shoulder joint is formed by the head of the humerus sitting in the socket of the scapula, seen here from the front (above) and the back (below).*

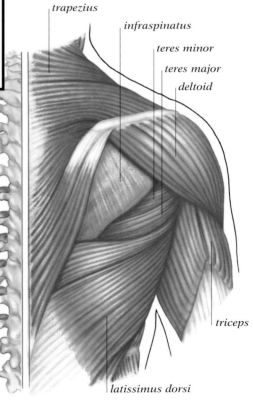

trapezius

infraspinatus

teres minor

teres major

deltoid

triceps

latissimus dorsi

Siamese twins

How common is it for Siamese twins to be born?

The birth of Siamese twins is extremely rare; probably only one pair are born in every 250,000 births. The few who survive tend to attract a great deal of publicity.

I know that some families have a higher chance of having twins. Is a woman who has had Siamese twins more likely to have another set?

A woman having more than one set of Siamese twins has never been recorded.

Has any pair of Siamese twins remained joined for life?

Most of the Siamese twins born in the past remained joined together for life. The most famous pair, Chang and Eng Bunker, who were born in Siam in 1811 (and who gave rise to the term "Siamese twins") are a notable example. They were exhibited as curiosities for many years, and later married and became farmers in America.

Is it difficult to operate on Siamese twins, and can they live a normal life once they are separated?

Whether it is possible to operate depends on the site and extent of the union between the twins. Certain Siamese twins have been successfully separated by surgery, particularly when they were joined only by skin or cartilage, or when the joined area was not extensive. When vital organs are shared, separation may be impossible.

Do Siamese twins occur only in humans?

No, they have been recorded in other species such as snakes, cattle, and sheep, but this is also extremely uncommon.

Siamese twins are twins who are born physically joined together, but have separate personalities. In the past, they remained conjoined, but with modern surgical advances they can be separated, although one or both may not survive.

Siamese twins got their name from the famous conjoined twins, Chang and Eng, who were born in 1811 to Chinese parents in Siam (now called Thailand). These twins, who were joined together at the abdomen, grew to a normal height and were able to walk, run, and swim. During their teens, the twins were taken to the United States by a British merchant, where they were displayed as curiosities. Later they were exhibited in Europe. They became American citizens, married English sisters, and fathered numerous children between them. After leaving show business, they became farmers in North Carolina, and died in 1874.

Chang and Eng, however, were by no means the first pair of conjoined twins. The first record of this phenomenon is of the Biddenden Maids, who were born in Kent, England, in medieval times. They were united from the shoulders to the hips, and had only one pair of arms and legs between them. Another set of twins who became famous were born in Italy in the 14th century

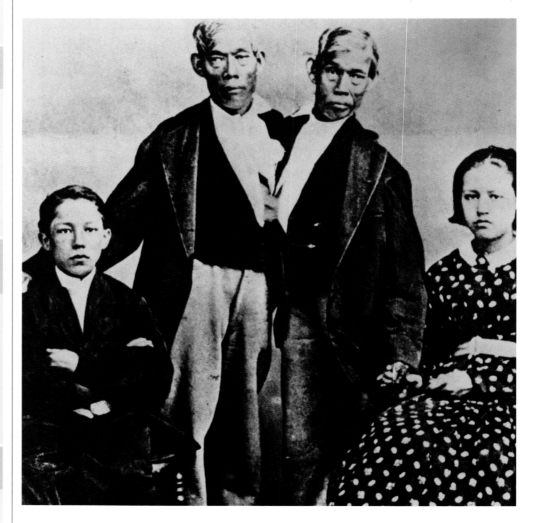

▲ *The term "Siamese twins" came from the famous pair Chang and Eng Bunker, who were born in Siam (Thailand). After a time in show business, they married two English sisters and fathered numerous children before they died at 63.*

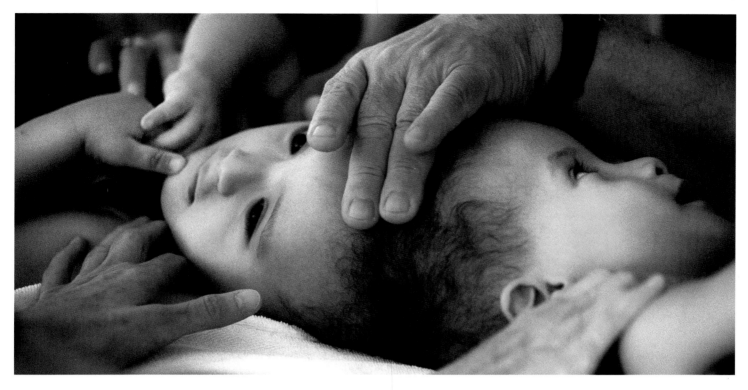

▲ *Egyptian Siamese twins Mohamed and Ahmed Ibrahim, joined at the top of their heads, were later successfully separated in an operation when they were two years old at the Children's Medical Hospital in Dallas, Texas, on October 12, 2003.*

and were known as the Florentine twins. They are the subject of a low relief in the Church of La Scala and of a sonnet. They had three arms and three legs between them.

Siamese twins may be joined at different parts of their bodies. They may be joined at the head, sternum (breastbone), chest, navel, pelvis, and back. Some are only joined superficially by skin or cartilage, but others share deeper vital organs, such as the heart or liver. In many this is incompatible with life, and they die at birth or soon afterward.

How Siamese twins occur

The birth of Siamese twins is an extremely rare occurrence. It is thought to occur in one in every 250,000 births.

When the ovum (egg) from a mother is fertilized by a sperm from the father, they form a cell called a zygote (see Conception). Usually this zygote develops to form one individual. In identical twins the zygote divides completely into two, and separate, though identical, individuals develop. (Nonidentical twins develop when two different ova are fertilized by two different sperm at the same time.)

It has been suggested that for Siamese twins to occur, rather than the zygote dividing in two it begins to develop into one person, and then at a slightly later stage of development (the precise time is unknown) it divides, but not completely. It is this incomplete separation that results in conjoined twins.

Delivery

It is not surprising that the delivery of these twins can be a problem. More surprising, however, is the fact that many of them are able to have a normal delivery. For example, there were Siamese twins born in Kano, Nigeria, some 30 years ago, who were joined from the lower sternum to the navel. Not only did they have a normal delivery; it was performed by a student midwife.

Surgical separation

Many Siamese twins have been successfully separated by surgery. Separation is desirable if each twin has a full complement of tissues and organs needed for a separate existence. Successful surgery is most likely when the union is only of skin and possibly cartilage; this may occur when the fusion is at the sternum or navel.

Many Siamese twins, however, share vital structures or organs, often in a complicated way, and therefore surgical separation is impossible. When they are joined extensively at the navel, there may be fusion of the stomach, intestines, or liver; or in those joined at the lower part of the back, the spinal cord may be fused.

The pair of Siamese twins from Kano, Nigeria, were brought to Britain for surgery. Externally they were joined from the lower sternum to the navel; internally their livers were fused, and needed to be separated surgically—a difficult procedure. One twin died unexpectedly following surgery, but the other made a satisfactory recovery and returned to live in Nigeria.

Ladan and Laleh Bijani, female Iranian Siamese twins, joined at the head, were not so lucky. In 2003 at the age of 29, having both attained law degrees, they chose to be surgically separated. This was achieved after a 53-hour operation. However, neither twin survived the surgery.

With modern surgical techniques, it is now possible to separate many babies who in the past had to stay joined together for life. When organs are shared, however, parents and surgeons may be faced with the very difficult decision as to whether one twin should be sacrificed in the interests of the other's survival. Such a choice may be the only alternative to the inevitable death of both.

See also: **Multiple birth**

Sick building syndrome

Questions and Answers

When my company moved to a new building, a coworker took mineral and vitamin supplements to avoid sick building syndrome. Should I do the same?

People who are low in essential vitamins and minerals may be more susceptible to chemical sensitivity (one of the major causes of sick building syndrome), since some of these nutrients are used by the body to detoxify harmful chemicals. Plenty of exercise, the avoidance of smoking, and a diet high in fruit and vegetables are needed for health maintenance in office and other indoor workers. Taking supplements indiscriminately, however, without medical advice, can be dangerous. Antioxidant vitamins C and E may help to deal with toxic substances, but since the exact cause of sick building syndrome is not always clear, there may be no rational basis for such treatment. Rather than making assumptions about the causes of the problem, those responsible should investigate and remove hazards.

When we got a new air-conditioning system in my office, many people complained of headaches and dizzy spells, but I was fine. Now I've started to ache and to feel nauseated. Could it be because I've had my apartment decorated?

Even if you didn't suffer symptoms before, the effort of dealing with the chemicals in your office could have depleted your body's defenses and it could well be the case that the chemicals emitted by the new paint at home have overloaded your detoxifying capacity. Try finding a way to reduce the total load of toxic chemicals, perhaps by increasing ventilation, ensuring that there are few plastic and foam materials around you, or staying elsewhere while the paintwork is fresh.

When new furnishings, foam insulation, or double glazing are introduced to a home or office, its occupants may find themselves suffering from a wide variety of illnesses. This effect, known as sick building syndrome, is thought to be caused by sensitivity to chemicals in the environment.

In the late 1970s, as a result of a drive for energy conservation, many new and old buildings in the United States were insulated with urea foam formaldehyde insulation (UFFI). Even buildings without UFFI had their windows sealed to conserve heat or air-conditioning. A lot of people living or working in such insulated and sealed buildings quickly developed symptoms ranging from headaches and lack of concentration to aching joints and respiratory problems. The illness was named "sick building syndrome," and the culprits identified were formaldehyde in the insulating material and other chemicals released into the air from synthetic carpets and furnishings, many of them odorless or scarcely detectable. Tightly sealing buildings to save energy consumption has the side effect of preventing these chemicals from escaping. Whereas a well-ventilated building might have a total exchange of air every few hours, this could take several days or even weeks in sealed buildings. As a result, higher levels of chemicals are absorbed into the bodies of the occupants, who are often unaware they have been exposed to them. A report by the World Health Organization estimates that sick building syndrome affects around a third of those in new or refurbished homes or offices.

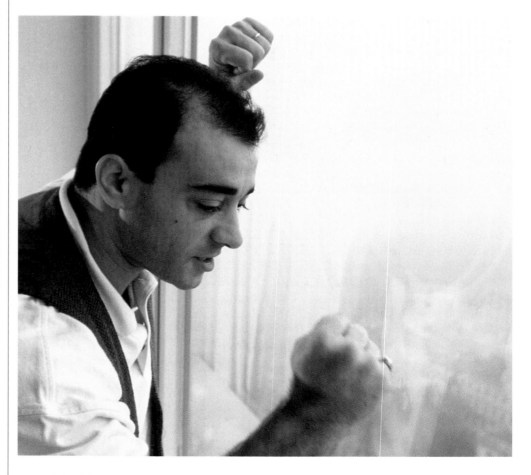

▲ *Sick building syndrome often occurs in tightly sealed buildings where poor ventilation promotes a potentially harmful buildup of chemicals.*

When people with the syndrome leave an environment that is causing the problem, or get rid of the offending furnishings, the illness sometimes clears up. For some people, however, it is not enough to avoid the original cause; they remain sick, and in a few cases get worse. The onset of sick building syndrome can promote sensitivity to other chemicals in the environment. The syndrome is often called environmental illness, a term that recognizes a wider range of causes other than a heavily insulated building.

The role of xenobiotics

The modern environment contains many chemicals that are foreign to our bodies, named "xenobiotics." Besides formaldehyde, these include chemicals present in foams, plastics, glues, and other materials used for building and furnishings: toluene, benzene, xylene, and styrene.

These xenobiotics are potentially toxic, but our bodies are normally well-equipped to break them down and get rid of them. However, the work of detoxifying the body consumes valuable nutrients and energy. When the body is deficient in the substances used to metabolize xenobiotics, or is faced with an overwhelming onslaught of toxic chemicals, the detoxification process may fail.

Symptoms of the syndrome

The symptoms that have been attributed to this chemical sensitivity vary widely. They may include joint pains, aching muscles, influenzalike aches, leg cramps, back pains, respiratory congestion or burning, abdominal pain, flushing, and a host of other seemingly unconnected ailments. Headaches and dizziness are common, as are all sorts of problems that are not physical, such as mood swings, depression, forgetfulness, or a spaced-out feeling.

There are a number of reasons for the enormous variety of symptoms. A huge variety of chemicals may be involved in sick building syndrome, each triggering different reactions. Some individuals may be less able to break down and get rid of particular xenobiotics, either because of some genetic factor or because of a nutritional deficiency. Another factor is the level of chemicals to which a sufferer has previously been exposed. It should not be assumed that all symptoms experienced by workers in such environments are necessarily attributable to sick building syndrome. Many of the health problems of office workers are caused by disorders, both physical and psychological, that have nothing to do with toxic chemicals.

Total load

If people are consistently exposed to one type of chemical—for example, from formaldehyde insulation in their home—their cells' metabolizing process will be constantly under strain, and their level of conjugated proteins will be low. Although these people may feel fairly healthy, even a relatively minor exposure to more chemicals, perhaps from solvents in the workplace, is likely to overload their detoxification capacity and result in chemical sensitivity. This phenomenon, called total load, helps to explain why only some occupants of a refurbished building suffer sick building syndrome.

Diet plays an important role in an individual's total load capacity. A diet high in processed foods is likely to be low in essential minerals, such as magnesium or zinc, that are vital constituents of the enzymes and conjugated proteins used in the detoxification process (see Diet).

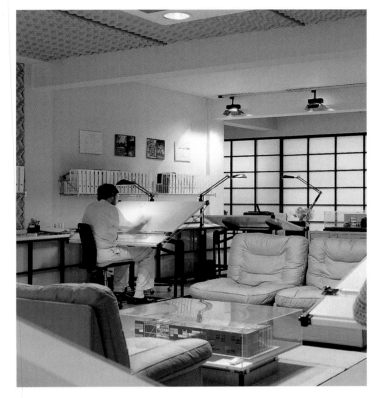

▲ *In new offices, synthetic furnishings and wall coverings can be potential sources of harmful xenobiotics.*

Diagnosis and treatment

The treatment for environmental illness should begin with a proper diagnosis. The sufferer should be asked for thorough details of home and work environments, leisure activities, and the pattern of symptoms in relation to his or her lifestyle. A patient who regularly wakes up with a headache, for example, may be exposed to a high level of xenobiotics in his or her bedroom.

The doctor should also take a medical and dental history. Although anesthesia is not obviously related to sick building syndrome, some patients start experiencing chemical sensitivity after they have been under anesthesia (see Anesthetics). Drugs, whether used to treat symptoms caused by sick building syndrome or by other diseases, may promote chemical sensitivity by reducing levels of nutrients needed for detoxification. Questions about the patient's diet may show up nutritional deficiencies that can easily be corrected.

The most effective treatment for sick building syndrome is to learn to reduce the total load. The sufferer is in the best position to do this by discovering what factors in his or her lifestyle promote the symptoms. It is often not enough simply to move away from the environment that seems to be causing the problem, even if this is possible. It may be helpful to change other aspects of a sufferer's environment—for example, someone who has been working in a tightly sealed building could replace synthetic furnishings at home with natural ones, so that exposure to xenobiotics is limited. Improving the diet by eating fresh foods, and cutting down the consumption of alcohol, can also make a significant difference.

See also: **Environmental hazards; Pollution; Vitamins**

Sickle-cell anemia

Sickle-cell anemia results from an abnormality in the hemoglobin, which is the oxygen-carrying pigment in the blood. It causes the red cells to distort into a sickle shape; it is a serious condition but can be controlled.

Questions and Answers

I have been told by my physician that I have a sickle-cell trait. Does this mean I could become anemic?

No, this is not a serious problem. The sickle-cell trait means that you have inherited from one parent a gene that gives rise to sickle-cell disease, but it is paired with a normal gene from your other parent. Although the abnormality can be seen in blood tests, it does not cause serious complications. Doctors may take extra care if you have anesthesia.

Are blood transfusions needed if someone has sickle-cell disease?

Possibly. One of the problems is that the red blood cells are very unstable and break down easily, causing anemia. It may be necessary to treat this with blood transfusions, particularly in pregnancy. However, exchange transfusions are given more often. A proportion of the patient's blood is removed and replaced with normal blood. This kind of treatment is used for sickle-cell crises, in which blood vessels have been blocked off by abnormal blood cells.

Is it true that there are many kinds of sickle-cell disease?

There is only one true kind of sickle-cell disease, in which the red blood cells carry the abnormal hemoglobin S, but there are some other abnormal hemoglobins that can cause problems. It is possible to inherit the genes for two different types of abnormal hemoglobin from your parents, leading to diseases in which both abnormalities are found.

The combination of hemoglobin S and another abnormal hemoglobin, C, is quite common, and is called SC disease. There are more than 300 kinds of abnormal hemoglobin, but only a few give rise to actual disease.

Each hemoglobin molecule is made up of a central heme portion, an iron compound responsible for carrying oxygen around the body, attached to which are four chains of globin molecules. The structure of the globin molecules determines that the hemoglobin will take up oxygen from the lungs and release it into the tissues where it is needed. Sickle-cell anemia results when abnormalities occur in the globin structure. The sickle cells are fragile and they are destroyed too quickly, so that the body tissues are deprived of oxygen.

This particular type of abnormal hemoglobin is called hemoglobin S and is distinct from normal hemoglobin A, which is found in the blood in large quantities after birth.

Causes

This abnormality is due to an abnormal gene inherited from both parents. Every characteristic in the body is controlled by a pair of genes (see Genetics), one of which is inherited from the mother and one from the father. In the case of hemoglobin, if you inherit one normal gene, the bone marrow will make a mixture of normal hemoglobin A and abnormal hemoglobin S. This is known as the sickle-cell trait (see Genetic Diseases and Disorders).

When both of the controlling genes are abnormal, the full-blown disease will result, and the red blood cells will contain a very high proportion of abnormal hemoglobin. People affected in this way are called homozygotes; those with only one abnormal gene are known as heterozygotes.

Sickle-cell disease is found in all parts of the world where

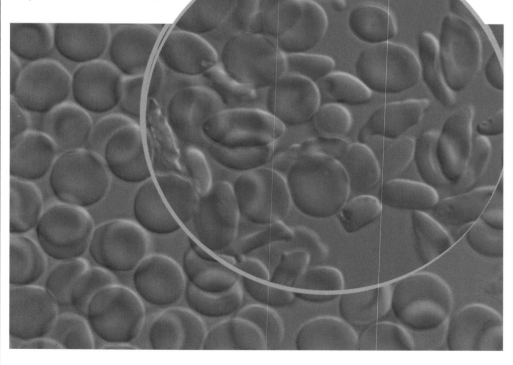

▲ *The blood cells in sickle-cell anemia twist into a characteristic sickle shape (inset), unlike the normal round cells of healthy blood.*

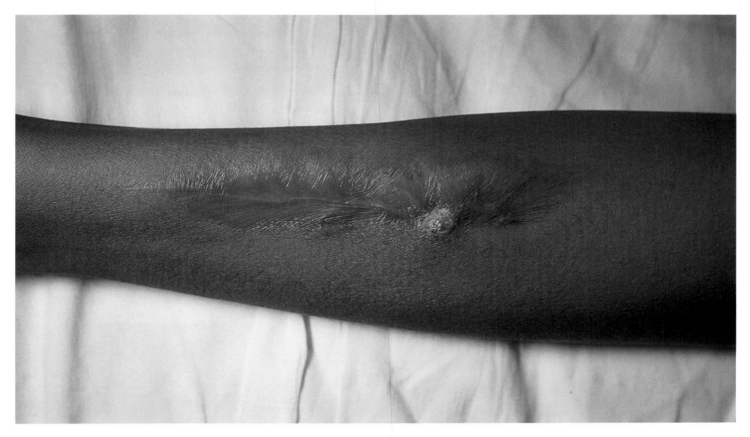

▲ *Abnormal cells in sickle-cell anemia can block and damage blood vessels throughout the body. This problem can lead to persistent leg ulcers as shown above.*

malaria is or has been prevalent (see Malaria) and so it is common in people of African origin. It has been estimated that one in 100 people of African descent suffer from sickle-cell anemia, and about one in 10 from sickle-cell trait.

The disease is also, but less commonly, found in Mediterranean regions, India, and western Asia. The inherited abnormality is thought to be so common because it gives protection against malaria. Because people with sickle trait were more likely to survive malaria in Africa than those who had normal hemoglobin, it is thought that this abnormal hemoglobin evolved as a protection against malaria. This, of course, is at the expense of those relatively few individuals who have the full-blown sickle-cell disease.

Symptoms

With homozygous sickle-cell disease, which results from two abnormal genes, the effects are extremely variable. In Africa, approximately 10 percent of children with the problem reach adult life. However, it is possible for the disease to be symptom-free and to be discovered only during routine blood tests (see Screening).

Chronic anemia can result from the continuous breakdown of red blood cells, but the greatest problem is the incidence of crises that occur when the oxygen level of the blood falls too low (see Blood). The hemoglobin molecules in the red cells then sickle or twist into an abnormal shape, making the cells twisted and stiff. These are known as sickle cells and give the disease its name. The deformed cells tend to accumulate and block off small blood vessels, make the

blood clot, and thus stop the tissues from receiving oxygen. Painful infarctions (areas of tissue that have died because of blocked circulation) then occur. The bones are often affected in this way. People with the sickle-cell trait may also be prone to crises under certain circumstances, such as during anesthesia (see Anesthetics).

The spleen can become enlarged as it separates abnormal cells from the blood. In time, infarction of the spleen will result so that it can no longer be felt in the abdomen. People with sickle-cell anemia are also more prone to infection, arising particularly from pneumococcus bacteria that cause lobar pneumonia. The disease also leads to leg ulcers.

Treatment

Treatment consists chiefly of treating the crises as they arise by rehydrating the patient with plenty of fluids and giving oxygen when necessary. It is also possible to give exchange transfusions so that abnormal sickle cells are replaced by normal blood (see Blood Transfusion).

Outlook

Improving methods of treating sickle-cell anemia have greatly increased the chance that those with the condition will survive into adulthood. Advances, too, have been made in preventing the disease through genetic counseling and by testing the blood of potential parents for the abnormal sickle-cell trait. Another preventive measure is to use amniocentesis to obtain and examine samples of fetal blood in early pregnancy, which makes it possible to detect any abnormality of the hemoglobin.

See also: **Anemia; Pain**

Side effects

Questions and Answers

My breasts enlarged when I took the Pill. Is this a side effect, and will they shrink when I stop taking it?

Yes they will. The Pill leads the body into thinking that it is pregnant. It contains normal female hormones of early pregnancy in smaller amounts than occur naturally, and this will produce some symptoms of pregnancy, such as swelling breasts or darkening of the nipples. These effects are now much less pronounced, because low-dosage pills are used.

If I start on a newly introduced drug, is there a chance that there will be unexpected side effects?

Yes. New drugs have to be tested very carefully—first on animals, then in controlled trials on patients. The licensing authority in the United States is the Food and Drug Administration, whose job is to decide whether a new drug is safe enough to be marketed. This decision will depend on whether the drug has any important advantages over similar existing drugs, but it is possible for side effects to occur even after a thorough testing period. In the case of a drug called practolol, widely used for treating angina, more than four years elapsed before it was realized that the drug was responsible for a rare form of fibrosis.

My son suffers badly from hay fever. Though antihistamines are a great help, they make him very sleepy. Can this be avoided?

There are other forms of treatment that do not cause sleepiness as a side effect. One approach is to use a nasal puffer that contains steroids in the hope of controlling the reaction. Some of the newer antihistamines are much less likely to cause your son to feel drowsy.

Many drugs can cause unwanted effects that may not be predictable or preventable. A doctor must weigh the benefits of a drug against the disadvantages of the side effects that may be produced.

Any drug taken can have "side effects," a term used to describe those secondary and usually undesirable effects that occur aside from the therapeutic purpose of the drug. Side effects can range from serious problems that require hospital treatment to minor difficulties that do not necessarily even require a change in dosage. There are many ways in which a drug can have unwanted effects. Sometimes the patient is simply oversensitive to the drug; in other cases there may be an abnormal response. An example of the latter is a rash that sometimes develops when penicillin is administered. Occasionally, the drug itself may have secondary effects that cannot be separated from its beneficial activity. Steroid drugs are a good example of this; the main reason for using them is to control the inflammatory response of the immune system, and when

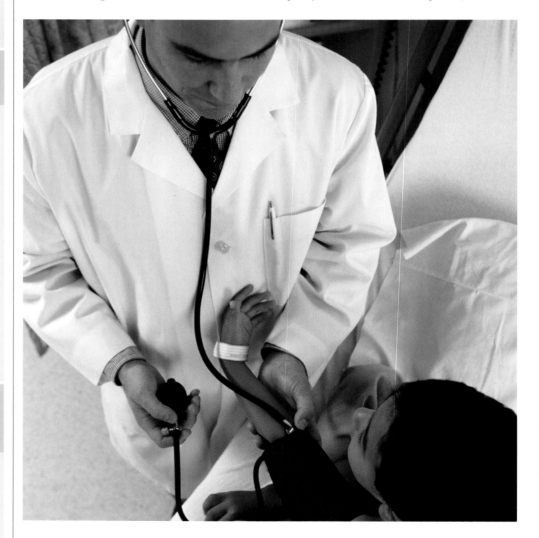

▲ *A doctor measures an injured child's blood pressure. Steroids may be necessary to control severe muscle inflammation after injury, but they can sometimes lead to high blood pressure, and patients must be carefully monitored. Children are particularly at risk from the side effects of steroids, since certain steroids are known to inhibit growth.*

they are taken they tend to cause the patient to put on weight.

Perhaps the most complex type of side effect occurs when two or more drugs are taken together and they interfere with each other. In recent years, as the range of drugs has widened, this problem has become more common and doctors are aware of it.

Drug dosage

For any drug to be effective, an appropriate dosage is essential that does not produce any toxic effects. If there is a large margin between an effective dosage and one that is toxic, the drug will be safe to use. However, a drug may have little margin between effective and toxic levels, in which case the drug is more difficult to use and doctors must control the dosage carefully. The margin between an effective dose and a toxic dose of a drug is known as the therapeutic index. Drugs with a very narrow therapeutic index are seldom used, unless they have desirable effects that cannot be achieved in any other way. Some anticancer drugs have a very narrow therapeutic index but are used because they are lifesavers.

The heart drug digitalis has been in use for 200 years, and for much of that time it was the only effective way of treating heart failure (see Heart Disease). Both digitalis and its modern derivative, digoxin, have narrow therapeutic indexes, and small doses can cause side effects such as vomiting and nausea. However, digoxin is safer to use, since it is possible to measure the level of the drug in the blood.

When two different drugs are given they may interact with each other and drug levels can easily build up in the body. This kind of

INTERACTION OF WARFARIN AND ASPIRIN

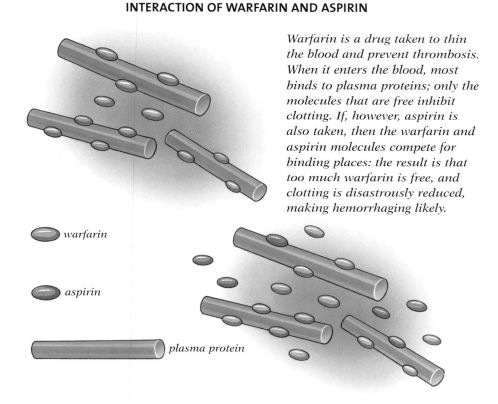

Warfarin is a drug taken to thin the blood and prevent thrombosis. When it enters the blood, most binds to plasma proteins; only the molecules that are free inhibit clotting. If, however, aspirin is also taken, then the warfarin and aspirin molecules compete for binding places: the result is that too much warfarin is free, and clotting is disastrously reduced, making hemorrhaging likely.

warfarin

aspirin

plasma protein

interaction occurs with warfarin, a blood-thinning drug used to prevent thrombosis and its complications (see Thrombosis). Warfarin prevents thrombosis by inhibiting normal clotting mechanisms; if there is an excessive amount of warfarin in the blood, clotting will not occur. Under normal circumstances warfarin is strongly bound to the plasma proteins, and only the small proportion of the drug that is free of its protein binding is actually active in stopping blood clotting. If, however, a patient on warfarin

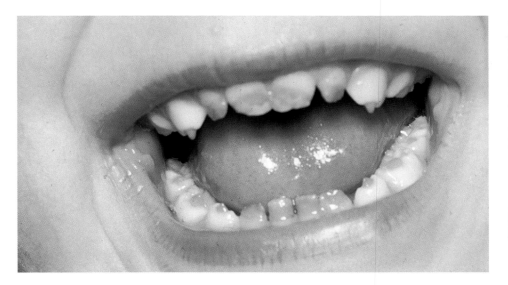

▲ *Tetracycline teeth are a possible side effect of the use of tetracycline. The condition takes the form of a darker-colored band of staining, usually across the middle of the teeth, that is extremely difficult to remove. Tetracycline was given often to children as an antibiotic in the 1960s and 1970s before this side effect was well known.*

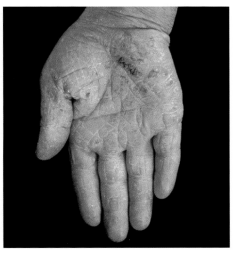

▲ *Some patients with heart trouble who were given the drug practolol developed eruptions on their hands. This, and other problems with the drug, led to its being withdrawn.*

takes another drug that is also bound to proteins, then more warfarin will be released into the blood as free, and therefore active, warfarin. This will seriously inhibit blood clotting. This happens because the two protein-bound drugs will compete with each other for the limited number of binding places, so that some warfarin is inevitably displaced. There are many drugs that will interact with warfarin in this way; aspirin is one example.

Kidney and liver failure

After a drug has been given to a patient, it is either excreted or changed by the body's metabolic processes. Many drugs are excreted by the kidneys in an active form. Therefore, in many patients who suffer a minor degree of kidney failure, the drug will be excreted at a rate lower than normal; and as a result toxic levels will build up in the bloodstream (see Kidneys and Kidney Diseases). Digoxin commonly causes toxicity when there is kidney failure, but almost any drug, including antibiotics, drugs to control blood pressure, and antidiabetic drugs, may give rise to trouble.

If a drug is not excreted by the kidneys, then it is nearly always excreted through the liver and bile system, often having been inactivated along the way. In the same way that minor degrees of kidney disease can lead to problems with toxicity in one group of drugs, so minor degrees of liver disease can lead to similar problems in other groups. The range of drugs affected by liver disease is small but still includes many widely used drugs, such as aminophylline, which is used in the treatment of asthma (see Asthma).

Age and the patient's condition

Aside from minor degrees of liver and kidney failure, there are many other ways in which a patient's state may affect the way that he or she responds to a particular drug; what would be a normal dose for a fit person produces undesirable side effects in someone in poor health. Many patients with respiratory problems are unable to take

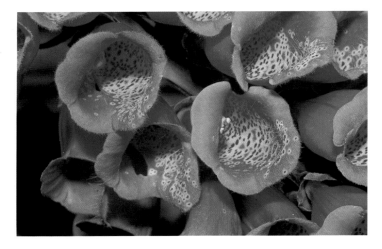

▲ *Foxglove is the source of the digitalis group of drugs, which are used to treat heart conditions. Digitalis has a narrow therapeutic index: even a fractional overdose will cause side effects such as loss of appetite, nausea, vomiting, and headache. The digitalis drug digoxin can sometimes disrupt normal heartbeat.*

any form of sedative or sleeping pill, since it may reduce the triggering of respiration. There is also a group of drugs that tend to make it difficult to urinate: antidepressants are a good example. People normally may not be affected, but an elderly man who has trouble with his prostate may be totally unable to urinate after a small dose of the drug. Prostate troubles are not the only way in which age interferes with the action of drugs. Elderly people can be unusually sensitive to a number of drugs, including sedatives and sleeping pills, and much smaller doses than usual should be taken.

Some side effects of drugs are related to recognized genetic (inherited) abnormalities. A hereditary disease called favism (a type of anemia, which occurs after eating a type of fava bean), has symptoms that also occur when people with the hereditary condition are given antimalarial treatment.

Porphyria is another inherited disease in which attacks may be set off by drugs. There are various manifestations of porphyria, but in one common form of the disease, abdominal pains are triggered by the use of contraceptive pills or barbiturates.

People vary in the way and the rate at which they metabolize drugs. In this instance, metabolism is the process by which the body absorbs and utilizes drugs, altering them and making them inactive.

One of the more common metabolic activities is a chemical process called acetylation. It has been found that most people acetylate drugs quickly, but some patients complete the process much more slowly. The tendency to be either a fast or a slow acetylator is inherited. Slow acetylators may experience side effects when taking the

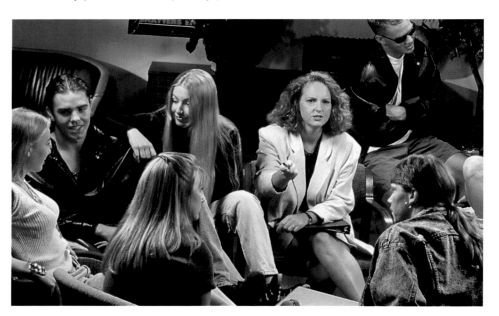

▲ *A drug rehabilitation session. Commonly abused drugs, including stimulants such as amphetamines, depressants such as alcohol, and narcotics such as cocaine, all have drug dependence as a side effect. Subsequent withdrawal often causes severe physical and psychological distress.*

Side effects of common drugs

DRUG	USE	SIDE EFFECTS
Antibiotics	To treat bacterial infection	May cause a rash, or upset the intestines by interfering with bacterial colonies usually found there
Anticoagulants	To thin the blood and prevent clotting	Excess activity may cause bleeding. Other drugs interfere with some anticoagulants—warfarin, for example, will be affected by alcohol.
Antihistamines	To treat symptoms of allergy: rash, hay fever	May cause sleepiness. It is dangerous to drive or to operate machinery while taking antihistamines.
Antidepressants	Treatment of depression	Can cause sleepiness, dry mouth, blurred vision, and difficulty in urination
Anticancer drugs	Treatment of all kinds of cancer	May block the formation of normal blood cells, leading to anemia and susceptibility to infection
Aspirin	A common painkiller	May cause indigestion and bleeding from the stomach and duodenum
Beta-blockers	Used in heart disease and high blood pressure to block the effect of adrenalin	May make patients feel tired and lethargic. Some people may suffer from cold hands and feet.
Diuretics	Used to treat heart failure, high blood pressure, and kidney disease	Can cause lack of potassium which can lead to muscle weakness and tiredness
Digoxin	To treat abnormal heart rhythms	May cause nausea and vomiting if dose is too large
Morphine	To treat severe pain	Vomiting is the main side effect, apart from morphine's being highly addictive. May also cause constipation.
Antipsychotic drugs	Treatment of serious psychiatric disease	May bring on symptoms of Parkinson's disease, which cease if drug is stopped
Steroids	Suppression of disease that results from overactivity of the immune system	Fluid retention leading to swelling; production of fat leading to weight increase. Muscles may get smaller. May produce high blood pressure.

antituberculosis drug isoniazid: the symptoms are abnormalities in function of the nerves of the skin, which in turn lead to numbness.

Drug allergy

Most of the side effects a doctor encounters are due to allergy. An allergy to a drug means that the body's immune system is activated by the drug, and it mounts an attack on the invader, which then shows up as a symptom—usually a skin rash, often accompanied by a fever (see Allergies). A response called anaphylaxis, or anaphylactic shock, is the most extreme form of drug allergy: a drug causes an almost immediate collapse, loss of blood pressure, wheezing, and a rash. Penicillin is the drug most likely to cause this reaction, although it is a rare problem. Anaphylaxis usually occurs only after injections rather than oral use of the offending drug, and responds well to treatment with epinephrine and other similar drugs. Many skin rashes are allergic, and there are few drugs that have never caused some sort of skin trouble. A rash may appear suddenly, or it may develop over a day or two (see Rashes).

The blood is also affected by many drugs, and the mechanism is usually through allergy and the production of abnormal antibodies by the immune system (see Immune System). In some cases the production of white blood cells is arrested by the drug, leaving the patient open to infection. Only a few drugs are likely to have this effect, which may be fatal, and it limits the drug's use. One such example is the antibiotic chloramphenicol, which is used only in the treatment of life-threatening infections such as typhoid.

Built-in side effects

The unwanted effects of a particular drug are often unavoidable, since they involve the way the drug works. Antibiotics may cause diarrhea by killing off the bacteria that normally inhabit the colon.

Steroid drugs have built-in side effects. Steroid hormones are part of the body's makeup, and have many effects on the body. When they are administered as a drug it is usually to control the activity of the immune system. However, steroids inhibit the manufacture of new protein as well as encouraging the body to make more fat. This leads to the characteristic moon face and weight gain of people on large doses of steroids, as well as loss of muscle bulk and thinning of the bones as a result of the loss of their basic protein structure, which is used as organic building material.

See also: **Shock; Steroids**

Sigmoidoscopy

Sigmoidoscopy is a valuable endoscopic procedure by which the whole of the inside of the rectum and lower part of the colon can be viewed. The procedure greatly increases the chances of detecting cancers at an early stage.

Questions and Answers

I am scheduled to have a sigmoidoscopy and I'm terrified of having a steel tube pushed into me. Is it going to be very painful?

No. The procedure doesn't require anesthesia, and it should be no more uncomfortable than using the toilet. Don't be alarmed at the sigmoidoscope's apparently large size. The outer opening of the anus is normally tightly closed and seems very small because of the muscle ring, the sphincter, surrounding it. When the muscle relaxes, the anal canal can easily widen to a greater diameter than the sigmoidoscope without undue stretching. The instrument is very smooth and highly polished, and a lubricant is used, so it glides easily.

I don't think I'll be able to relax. Could I be given a sedative?

Certainly, if the doctor thinks that it is necessary. However, you don't need a sedative to do what is the equivalent of an everyday process.

Surely I'll have pain as the sigmoidoscope moves about inside my intestine?

No. At most, you'll have a slight feeling of discomfort. The doctor will give you a manual examination to confirm that there are no obstructions to the passage of the sigmoidoscope. If you have any painful anal fissures or piles, local anesthesia will be used to make the procedure entirely painless. Just take it easy and you'll be all right.

I have to have a sigmoidoscopy and know I will be horribly embarrassed. How can I avoid this?

You needn't be. The doctor has done this hundreds of times and thinks nothing of it. He or she is interested only in what can be found. So if the doctor is not embarrassed, why should you be?

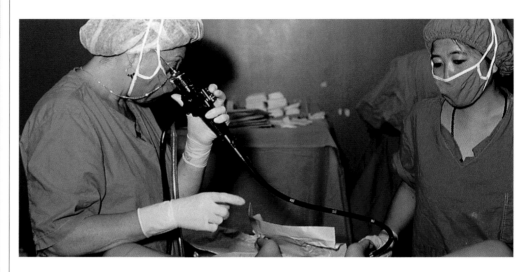

▲ *Sigmoidoscopy does not require admission to a hospital and can be done in a doctor's office. It seldom takes longer than half an hour and causes very little, if any, discomfort.*

The large intestine, or colon, which is suspended around the periphery of the inside of the abdominal cavity, descends on the left side and then makes an "s" (see Colon and Colitis). This is the sigmoid colon (*sigma* is the Greek letter "s"). Sigmoidoscopy is a direct visual examination of the inside of this part of the intestine, using an instrument called a sigmoidoscope—a flexible tube that contains fiber-optic channels to illuminate and view the inside of the colon and rectum.

Reasons for a sigmoidoscopy

Diseases of the lower intestine are very common, and it is often difficult, without direct inspection, to distinguish between them. Direct examination of the lining of the sigmoid colon and rectum is an invaluable aid in this task. Doctors familiar with the appearances of the interior of the intestine can at once distinguish such abnormalities as malignant and benign tumors and inflammation, and the presence of blood, pus, and other discharges (see Tumors). In many cases, biopsy specimens or scrapings of ulcers are taken for microscopic examination (see Ulcers).

However, the main reason for performing sigmoidoscopy is to detect or eliminate cancer of the intestine (see Cancer). Lower intestinal cancer is one of the most common forms of cancer, second only to lung cancer as a cause of cancer death in the United States, and its incidence has not changed much in the last 50 years. Any procedure that makes its diagnosis easier is thus very important. Sigmoidoscopy is also a valuable screening procedure for people with a family history of multiple intestinal polyps, who are especially susceptible to cancer. Many doctors believe that sigmoidoscopy should be performed routinely as a screening procedure on people over 40, especially if there is a family history of intestinal cancer.

In addition to lower intestinal cancer, there are other disorders that can be readily diagnosed by sigmoidoscopy. Examples include Crohn's disease, an inflammatory intestinal disorder that affects the wall of the colon; polyps, which are button-mushroomlike benign growths on the lining of the intestine; inflammation of the rectum and anal canal (proctitis); and internal piles (see Anus; Hemorrhoids).

> *See also:* Biopsy; Crohn's disease; Endoscopy; Polyps; Rectum

Silicosis

Questions and Answers

I have worked with sandblasting machinery for two years. Are my chances of getting silicosis high?

No. The use of sand or other materials containing silica is prohibited by law, and relatively harmless substitutes are used.

Is there a connection between silicosis and tuberculosis (TB)?

In the 1930s both silicosis and TB were common among ordinary workers, and it was not unusual for both diseases to occur together. Also, there did seem to be an extra predisposition to TB in silicosis sufferers. TB still occurs under certain circumstances, but is less likely to occur in people who risk contracting silicosis.

My son is training to become a stonemason. I am worried that he might get silicosis. Is this likely?

No. Silicosis is no longer a serious problem among stonemasons. However, stringent precautions need to be taken when dealing with such stones as granite and sandstone. Precautions include using water when cutting the stones, to dampen the dust, and wearing breathing apparatus.

Is it true that some people are more at risk of silicosis?

Yes. Miners have developed silicosis after being employed for only a few months drilling rock with a high silica content, while others have carried out similar work for up to 30 years with no ill effects. No explanations have been given for these differences. Those people who expend more energy will breathe particles more deeply into their lungs and face greater risks; those with previous lung disease, and smokers, with diminished ciliary action, are said to be more susceptible to silicosis.

Of all the occupational lung diseases caused by dust, silicosis is the most common and serious. Once it is established, there is no cure, so prevention is essential to reduce the amount of silica dust that is inhaled.

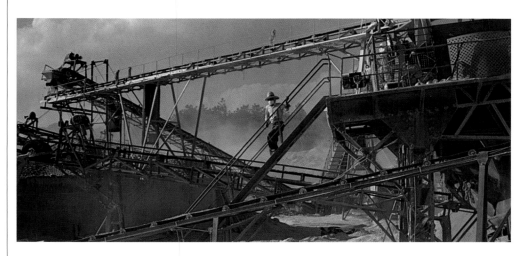

▲ *A quarry worker in Okinawa, Japan, wears a protective mask which prevents him from inhaling particles of dust that could otherwise cause silicosis.*

Silicosis is a serious lung disease caused by inhaling dust particles of free silica—a substance found in stones such as quartz, granite, sandstone, and flint. Very small silica particles reach the lung alveoli where they are taken up by large phagocytes (macrophages). Silica is toxic to these cells and kills them, releasing the protein-splitting enzymes used by the macrophages, and freeing the silica particles. The enzymes break up local tissues and the healing causes scarring (fibrosis). The released silica particles are then taken up by other macrophages and the cycle repeats. At the present time, however, with improved protection and the increased use of safe substitute materials, silicosis is a far rarer disease than it once was, although mining continues to be a common cause of exposure to silica (see Lung and Lung Diseases).

In sandblasting, for instance (an occupation traditionally linked with silicosis), the use of sand is now prohibited. Comparatively safe substitutes have been found in corundum or silicon carbide. Silicosis is also no longer a problem for stonemasons. When dealing with siliceous stones, they use water to dampen the dust, and they wear breathing protection. Despite stringent dust controls, the danger of silicosis still lurks in the pottery industry. The main hazard here is the ground flint used to improve the clay. Substitutes such as a mixture of quartz and cristobalite are now used, but these materials also contain silica. A safer alternative, alumina, is too expensive for general use.

Silicosis causes nodular fibrosis of the lungs. The symptoms follow three stages. First, the victim gets breathless with an unproductive cough. Second, breathlessness becomes worse and physical exertion is difficult. Third, the victim is incapacitated and suffers fatigue, loss of weight, productive cough, chest pain, and severe breathlessness. However, before these symptoms appear and serious damage has been done to the lungs, silicosis can and should be diagnosed by taking X rays. If this is done early enough and the cause of the disease removed, the silicosis need not be progressive. If the condition is allowed to progress, the lungs will fail to absorb enough oxygen for the blood, and heart failure can occur (see Breathing; Chest; Heart).

There is no cure for silicosis, so it is vital to prevent exposure to silica by finding safe substitutes, by controlling the dust through effective exhaust ventilation or by the use of protective clothing; in some cases this may require a suit with its own air supply.

See also: Environmental hazards

Sinusitis

Sinusitis, or inflammation of the air cavities in the bones around the nose, is a common problem. It can cause considerable discomfort but most cases are treated successfully.

The sinuses are small cavities in the bones of the face. They contain air, thus contributing to the skull's lightness. The sinus cavities are linked with the nose and the upper throat, and are therefore vulnerable to the spread of infection from these areas. The condition can be divided into acute sinusitis and chronic sinusitis; each has different symptoms. Children under the age of five rarely suffer from sinusitis, because their sinuses are not yet fully developed.

Causes

The nose and sinuses are lined with special cells that produce mucus to combat any initial infections, for example, from a cold or influenza virus. When a virus enters the body, mucus production increases, which makes the lining of the nose and sinuses swell, and blocks up the communicating channels between them. The mucus can no longer escape, pressure builds up, and the infection in the sinuses is trapped. Bacteria that normally live in the nose and sinuses now multiply and the sinuses become filled with yellow or green pus (see Pus).

It is this pus which, being under pressure, creates the symptoms of sinusitis. Allergies are also commonly associated with sinusitis (see Allergies). Dental infections, fractures of the facial bones, or gunshot wounds may also lead to sinusitis. Poor drainage of the nose and enlarged, infected adenoids and tonsils are also factors contributing to this condition.

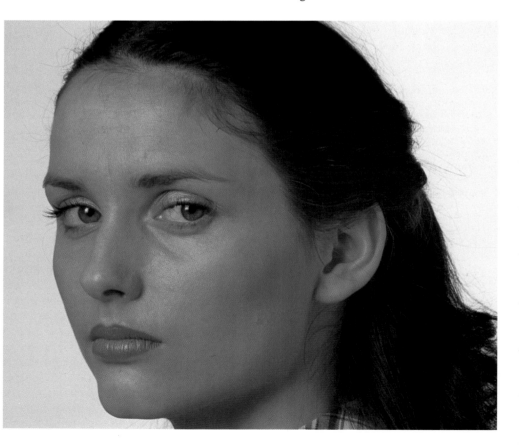

▲ *In an attack of sinusitis, pain may be felt in the forehead, behind the eyes and nose, at the back of the head or neck, or beneath the eyes.*

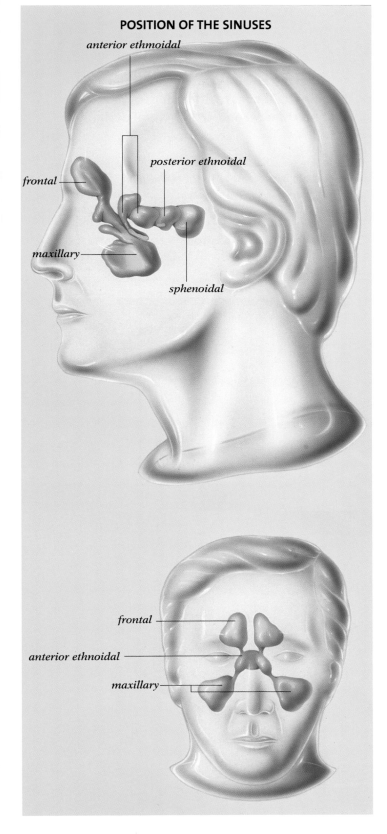

POSITION OF THE SINUSES

anterior ethmoidal

posterior ethnoidal

frontal

maxillary

sphenoidal

frontal

anterior ethnoidal

maxillary

▲ *The sinus cavities in the skull are interconnected, and they all open into the nasal cavity. Therefore, infection can easily spread from the nose to involve any of these mucus-producing cavities.*

Symptoms and dangers

Acute sinusitis gives rise to pain and sometimes redness and swelling over the sinus. The patient may have a severe localized headache, depending on which sinus is affected. Frontal sinusitis, for example, produces pain above the eyes. In maxillary sinusitis, there is pain in the cheeks, which is often throbbing and is made worse by bending down or by moving the head. The nose is blocked on the affected side, but there may be very little discharge. The senses of smell and taste are usually reduced.

Chronic sinusitis produces nasal discharge, low-grade pain, a blocked nose, and cough, and in children there may be a tendency to get ear infections. The infection continues for weeks or months, and often follows an acute initial infection. Sometimes infection of one of the frontal sinuses spreads around the eye, causing double vision, swelling of the eyelids, or even an abscess behind the eyeball which pushes it outward. Meningitis or a brain abscess may also develop.

Middle-ear infections often occur with maxillary sinusitis and, in children, can sometimes result in deafness (see Otitis). An infection in the ear may also spread downward and cause conditions such as laryngitis or pneumonia.

Treatment

It is important to treat sinusitis and all related infections thoroughly to prevent the development of possible serious complications.

An X ray may be taken to locate trapped fluid. Polyps, which are overgrowths of the mucous membrane lining the nose, may be present (see Polyps). Acute sinusitis is treated with antibiotics, decongestant nose drops perhaps containing ephedrine, menthol inhalations, and painkillers. Steam inhalations can help to clear the nose and relieve the symptoms.

In some cases of sinusitis it may be necessary to drain out the pus from the sinus through a small hole made on the inside of the nose. Surgery may also be of use in chronic sinusitis or when there are polyps. In children with sinusitis it is often best to remove the adenoids and tonsils. Washing out the sinuses with a saltwater (saline) solution can also be helpful after pus has been drained off.

Outlook

Sinusitis can be difficult to treat once a chronic condition has become established, and each ensuing infection can cause a more stubborn chronic infection than the previous infection. Unduly vigorous nose blowing should be avoided; this can force infected material into the sinuses. Nose drops and sprays should not be used for more than a week at a time because they can create further problems; they are of value only in short courses. Antibiotics help to cure infection, but, since they are absorbed into the bloodstream, it is difficult for them to work within a sinus where there is no blood supply. Acute sinusitis often clears up with antibiotics and nose drops. Chronic sinusitis, however, may last a long time, especially if the sufferer is a heavy smoker. A nasal tumor should be ruled out in cases of chronic sinusitis. Sinusitis is more common in the winter, partly because there are more germs that cause upper respiratory infections at that time of the year. A sufferer may be free of symptoms in the summer but spend the winter having to deal with a blocked nose and low-grade pain. Serious complications following a bout of sinusitis appear to be rare.

See also: **Deafness; Hearing**

Skeleton

Questions and Answers

How much force is needed to break a bone?

It varies according to the position, shape, and health of the bone. The long thin bones of the arms and legs are more prone to snapping fractures than are the plate bones of the shoulder and pelvis, which are more prone to heavy blows or crushing injuries. People who are undernourished, and older people whose bones have lost part of their protein framework, have brittle bones that break easily. Generally, however, it is amazing how much force a bone can withstand.

What is a greenstick fracture?

In this type of fracture, instead of the bone breaking into two or more separate fragments, only one side of it actually breaks. The other side is more bent than broken. The appearance and effect are similar to what happens if you try to break a stick of wood that is still green, hence the name. These fractures usually occur only in children whose bones have not yet fully ossified and are thus more supple.

Do bones ever just give way and break by themselves?

Yes, though a much more common situation is that the bone is exposed to some stress or injury, but to a lesser degree than would usually be required to break it. These are called spontaneous fractures and result from the bones' being thinner and weaker than normal, usually because of an inadequate diet or some hormonal or metabolic upset that interferes with the normal hardening or ossification process. Also, some diseases remove protein or calcium from the bones, weakening the bones and making them more prone to breakage, in which case a fracture is called pathological. Bones invaded by a tumor may also fracture spontaneously.

Strong enough to protect the vital organs, intricately structured to keep the body upright, and flexible enough to allow great freedom of movement, the human skeleton is a marvel of mechanical and architectural design.

The skeleton of the average adult is made up of 206 bones, though there may be variation in the number of ribs, an additional pair occasionally occuring in the neck. The bones have a hard, thick, strong outer layer and a soft middle, or marrow (see Marrow and Transplants). They are as strong and as tough as concrete and can support great weights without bending, breaking, or being crushed. Linked together by joints and moved by muscles that are attached at either end (see Muscles), they provide cages to protect the soft and delicate parts of the body while still allowing for great flexibility of movement. In addition, the skeleton is the framework or scaffolding on which the other parts of the body are hung and supported.

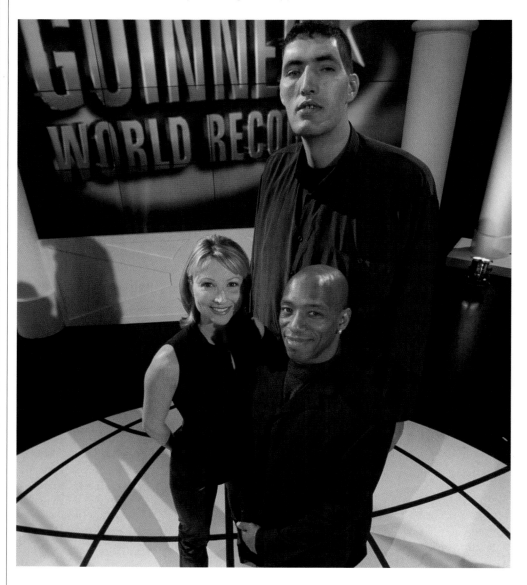

▲ *The skeleton can adapt itself to a large range of sizes, as shown in this photo shoot for 1999's Guinness World Records' tallest man, Rhadouane Charbib (center).*

Men and women have the same number of bones, but in general the female skeleton is lighter and smaller. In order to accommodate the growing fetus during pregnancy, a woman's pelvis (right) is broader and more boat-shaped, giving her hips their characteristic shape. Her shoulders, however, are relatively narrow. In a man (left), the proportions are reversed: broad shoulders and slim hips.

Questions and Answers

Is cartilage another type of bone tissue?

Strictly speaking, cartilage and bone are distinct types of tissue, although they have strong similarities. Bone is cartilage that has been hardened by the deposition of mineral salts so that it becomes tougher and can withstand much greater wear and tear. In parts of the body where a slightly softer and more flexible substance than bone is required, the skeleton consists of cartilage; the tip of the nose and the cushioning disks between the bones of the spine are examples.

I have heard references to the musculoskeletal system. What is it?

In its medical sense, a system is made up of all the parts or tissues and organs in the body that act together to produce a particular effect or that participate in a particular process. The bones of the skeleton exist not on their own but in conjunction with other supporting and connective tissues such as ligaments, and in particular muscles, through which movement is made possible. It is thus more sensible, in terms of function, to think of the skeleton and muscles together rather than separately.

Is the skeleton susceptible to cancer?

Yes, it is; but this is not very common. In most cases, the cancer does not start in the bone itself, but is carried there through the blood supply from a primary site elsewhere in the body. The cancer cells may then become established in the bone and form a secondary growth. There are two main types of cancer that start in the bone, though these are rare. The first is called an osteogenic sarcoma and usually occurs in one of the long bones, such as the femur or the tibia, of a teenager. The other, called multiple myelomatosis, starts in several different bones (the ribs, vertebrae, skull, and pelvis being the most common) and interferes with the blood-forming marrow.

Structure of the skeleton

Each of the different parts of the skeleton is designed to do a particular job. The skull protects the brain, eyes, and ears. The lower jaw and teeth are attached to it, enabling us to eat. There are holes for the eyes, ears, nose, and mouth, and also one in the base of the skull where it joins the spinal column; the spinal cord passes through this, connecting the brain to the rest of the body.

The backbone, or spine, is made up of a chain of small bones, similar to spools of thread, called vertebrae, and forms the central axis of the skeleton. It has enormous strength, but, because it is a rod made up of small sections, instead of being one solid piece of bone, it is also very flexible. This enables people to bend down and touch their toes, and to hold themselves stiff and upright. The vertebrae also protect the delicate spinal cord. Between the vertebrae are shock-absorbing disks that act as cushions to help protect the vertebrae from rubbing on each other and becoming damaged as a person bends down and straightens up. The bottom end of the spinal column is called the coccyx. In some animals, such as the dog and cat, this forms a tail.

The rib cage is made up of the ribs at the sides, the spinal column at the back, and the breastbone, or sternum, in front. It is designed to protect the heart and lungs that lie inside it, since damage to these organs could prove fatal.

The arms are joined onto the central axis of the spinal column by the shoulder girdle, which is made up of the scapula (shoulder blade) and the clavicle (collarbone). The big bone of the

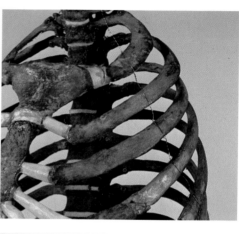

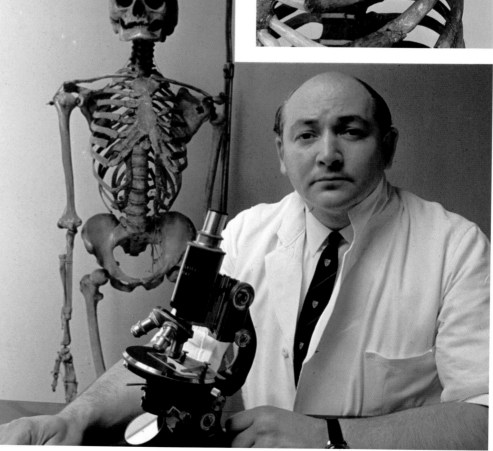

▲ *Forensic pathologists sometimes reconstruct skeletal remains to establish the cause of a violent death. The inset shows the rib cage of a woman who was buried for five years in a shallow grave: the fourth and fifth ribs are fractured—injuries due to a knife thrust.*

upper arm (the humerus) is joined at the elbow to the two bones of the forearm: the radius and ulna (see Elbow). The hand is made up of many small bones. This makes it possible for people to grip things and to make delicate, complicated movements in which each of the many parts of the hand moves in a different yet highly coordinated way.

The legs are attached to the spine by the pelvic girdle, which shields the reproductive organs and the bladder and gives protection to the developing baby which lies in this part of its mother's body. The femur (the thick bone of the thigh) is the longest bone in the body. Its round head fits into the socket in the pelvis to form the hip joint, which is designed to maximize freedom of movement of the leg (see Hip). There are two bones in the lower leg: the shinbone, or tibia, and the much thinner fibula.

The foot, like the hand, is made up of a complicated arrangement of small bones. This enables people both to stand firmly and comfortably and to walk and run without falling over.

How the skeleton develops

Surprising as it may seem, a newborn baby has more bones in its body than an adult. At birth, around 350 bones make up the tiny frame; over the years some of these fuse together into larger units.

A baby's skull is a good example of this; during the birth process, it is squeezed through a narrow canal. Were the skull as inflexible as an adult's it would simply not be possible for the baby to pass through the mother's pelvic outlet. The fontanelles, or gaps between the sections of the skull, allow it to be molded sufficiently to accommodate itself to the birth canal. After birth, these fontanelles gradually close.

The skeleton of a child is made not only of bone, but also of cartilage, which is much more flexible. Gradually this hardens into bone—a process known as ossification, which continues well into adulthood. It is not until the age of about 20 that full skeletal maturity is reached.

The proportions of the human skeleton change dramatically as people mature. The head of a six-week-old embryo is as long as its body; at birth the head is still large in proportion to the body, but the midpoint has shifted from the baby's chin to the navel. Each person has his or her own timetable for skeletal growth, but it can be affected by such environmental factors as diet and disease. Certain glandular disorders can cause too much or too little growth; rickets is caused by a lack of vitamin D (see Rickets). Sometimes people are born with extra bones, such as an extra pair of ribs. In general, the frame of a woman is lighter and smaller than that of a man's. Her pelvis is proportionately wider, and it allows room for the growing fetus during pregnancy. The male shoulders are broader and the rib cage is longer but, contrary to popular superstition, men and women have the same number of ribs.

Evolution

About 25 million to 30 million years ago the primates (the subgroup of mammals to which humans belong) abandoned the trees which had been their habitat and took to terrestrial life. At this stage they probably walked on all four limbs. They relied on the sense of sight rather than smell and so the eye sockets were forward-looking and both hands and feet had the ability to grasp. Gradually, through evolution, the feet of these human ancestors became specialized: the ability to cling to branches was no longer needed. As humans began to walk upright, the foot had to be adapted to take the forces brought to bear on it: the fingers grew longer, the toes remained short and the big toe became nonopposable, that is, it could no longer be placed in opposition to the others, as the thumb can be to the other fingers. The heel has to come into contact with the ground at the beginning of the stride and the weight of the body is transferred over the arch to the big toe, which has to be in line with the direction of movement.

Some six million years ago our predecessor *Australopithecus*, though a biped, looked startlingly different from humans today. The bones of the skull were

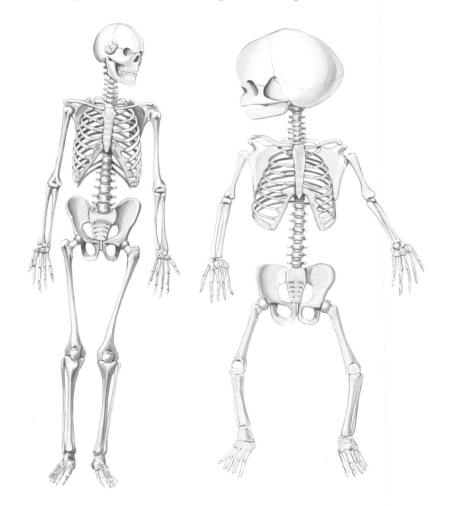

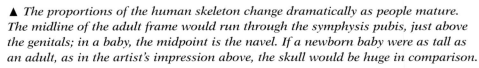

▲ *The proportions of the human skeleton change dramatically as people mature. The midline of the adult frame would run through the symphysis pubis, just above the genitals; in a baby, the midpoint is the navel. If a newborn baby were as tall as an adult, as in the artist's impression above, the skull would be huge in comparison.*

EVOLUTION OF THE FOOT

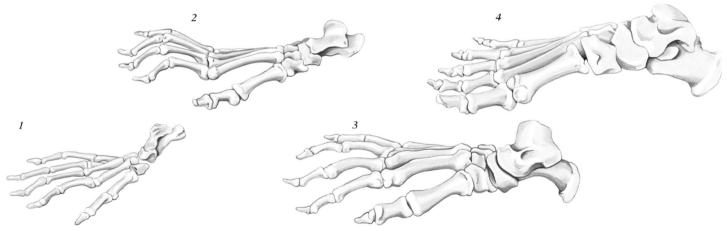

more massive; *Australopithecus* had a larger facial area, more prominent brow ridges, a flatter crown, and a smaller braincase. The gait was stooping, the legs were comparatively short, and the arms were comparatively long. Height was only about 4 feet (approximately 1.25 m). As these anthropoid primates evolved to become more like modern humans, and as they developed a more striding gait, the legs grew longer and the pelvis narrower. The fact that humans have developed great manual dexterity, however, is due less to skeletal sophistication (the hands are primitive adaptations from the fins of amphibious ancestors) than to the increasing capacity of a human's brain. In strictly anatomical terms, the human hand differs little from that of the apes, the relatives of humans.

The human skeleton of today is the result of millions of years of evolution, designed to equip it for the complex tasks it must perform. Questions such as whether the evolutionary process is complete, and whether the skeleton will develop further, and, if so, how, are the stuff of science fiction, not medicine. What modern medicine can ensure is that the injuries and disease to which our internal scaffolding is subject become better understood and more easily treated.

What can go wrong?

While the bones of the skeleton are very resilient, if the weight or pressure on them becomes too great they will break. A bone may break from being crushed, from a sharp impact on its middle, or from force at one end causing it to snap. The amount of force required to break a bone varies with the individual: older people, whose bones are thinner and less resilient, are more prone to fractures. Treatment depends on the severity and position of the break, but involves ensuring that the broken bone is held together in the right position until the damaged ends grow together again (see Fractures; Orthopedics).

Though the spine usually functions without trouble, it is hardly surprising that something in the long pile of vertebrae on their disks, rather precariously balanced one on top of the other, occasionally slips out of place (see Slipped Disk). Sometimes the vertebrae become displaced; this is called spondylolisthesis and occurs most commonly in the lower back, or lumbar, region. At other times, one of the disks cushioning the vertebrae slips to become a prolapsed intervertebral disk. Rest and physical therapy are the best treatment for this condition (see Back and Backache; Physical Therapy). The spine is also prone to degenerative disorders (which are usually

▲ *Human evolution has involved many changes to the skeleton, including the foot. In humans' tree-living ancestors, the toes were long and the big toe could be opposed to the others (1, 2). Then an upright posture was adopted (3), and eventually humans developed a striding walk. The ability to grasp has been lost; the big toe is in line with the others and is large because it has to take much of the force of each step (4).*

brought about by aging) and can also become temporarily deformed by being held in abnormal positions when a patient is trying to avoid pain. The hunchback type of deformity is called kyphosis; forward curvature is called lordosis, and sideways curvature, scoliosis (see Aging; Scoliosis).

Osteoporosis, a bone disorder, affects many postmenopausal women (who have lost the anabolic effect of estrogen) and whose bones have become weakened by loss of both the protein (collagen) structure and the calcium and phosphate mineralization (see Calcium; Protein). Osteoporosis leads to pathological fractures from minor trauma, especially of the arm, spine, and neck of the femur, and is responsible for an immense amount of suffering, disfigurement, and disablement in older women (see Osteoporosis).

Joints

The skeleton is a highly articulated piece of machinery. The many finger joints allow people to grasp objects; the elbow enables them to lift objects up; the knees ensure that they are able to walk, run, jump, and so on (see Knee). The joints themselves are lined with lubricated cartilage, so the bone ends do not rub against one another; if the cartilage gets worn away, as in cases of osteoarthritis, pain and stiffness result (see Osteoarthritis). The bone may try to compensate for the subsequent damage by repairing itself. This bone growth is haphazard, however, and can lead to skeletal deformity: many people with arthritic finger joints, for example, develop extra knobs of bone known as Heberden's nodes (see Arthritis). Overuse of certain joints can lead to tennis elbow or frozen shoulder (see Tennis Elbow).

Heat, gentle exercise, and occasionally injections of hydrocortisone and local painkillers can help (see Exercise; Heat Treatment).

See also: **Bones; Cartilage; Feet; Hand; Joints; Neck; Pelvis; Ribs; Shoulder; Spinal cord**

Skin and skin diseases

Questions and Answers

Why are skin conditions so often inflamed by emotional upsets?

Most ill health is made worse by emotional upsets, and the skin is no exception. Emotion can also alter the state of the skin's irritability and sweating mechanisms. Conditions in which these factors are important, such as eczema, will be aggravated by anxiety, discontent, or depression.

I have developed an allergy to nickel because I wore cheap jewelry. Will I always be allergic?

Allergy to nickel is fairly common in those who either wear or handle it. There is always an interval between first contact with nickel and the development of the allergy. Traces of nickel are absorbed through the skin and the body reacts by forming antibodies so that any further contact results in an itchy skin rash. If no further contact occurs the allergy will gradually lessen. However, it usually remains to some degree throughout life.

I have bald patches on my scalp and beard area. Will they regrow?

Bald patches are a symptom of a condition called alopecia areata, which may run in families and frequently starts in childhood. Hair is lost in clear-cut round areas, often a few weeks after stress or shock. It usually calms down, and in most cases hair regrows in two to six months, although relapses are common.

My husband is 20 and is going bald. Is this normal?

Yes. Hair loss in men may begin at any time after puberty as a result of higher male hormone levels. Often there is a hereditary factor as well. The drug minoxidil (Rogaine), used locally under medical supervision, can aid hair regrowth.

The skin is the largest human organ, although it is not often thought of as such. It protects people from injury and infection, as well as keeping the body's temperature and moisture content stable at all times.

The skin is much more than a simple wrapping for the body. It is an active and versatile organ that is waterproof so that people do not dry up in the heat or dissolve in the rain, and it protects them from the damaging radiation of sunlight. It is tough enough to act as a shield against injury, yet supple enough to permit movement. It conserves heat or cools the body as required, thereby keeping the internal temperature constant.

Skin diseases may be a nuisance and cause embarrassment, but they are seldom dangerous and are rarely fatal. However, they can cause a lot of ill health by their very frequency and persistence.

Structure of the skin

The skin has two main parts. The outermost part, the epidermis, consists of several layers of cells, the lowest of which are called the basal cells, or mother cells. These cells are constantly dividing and the offspring cells are pushed up to the surface by subsequent offspring cells, where they progressively flatten as they approach the surface. The surface cells eventually die and are

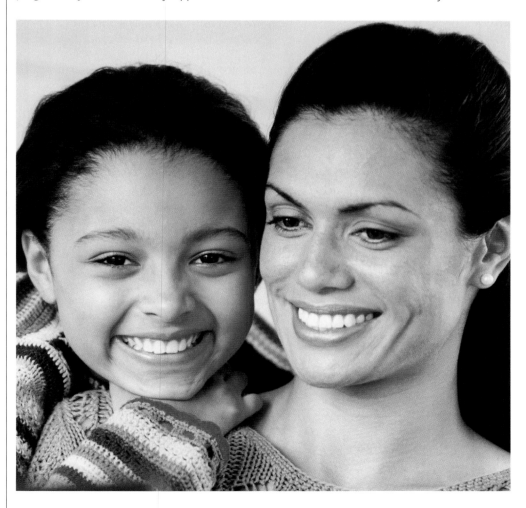

▲ *A person's skin type and his or her coloring are determined by heredity. Hair and nails are formed from skin cells, and these too are determined by genetic factors.*

Why does some people's skin age faster than others?

Inheritance is probably the most important factor in skin aging. Other influences involved are the environment, such as the amount of sun damage and hormonal changes throughout life. The loss of elasticity that causes wrinkles in old age is due to changes in the fibers of the supporting layer of skin. Skin also becomes drier and hair thinner with age.

Do commercial suntanning preparations really prevent burning and promote a suntan?

There are suntanning preparations that claim to prevent sunburn and enhance tanning. This can only happen with an efficient sunscreen, which enables you to sunbathe for longer periods, and builds up the protective pigmentation so that a gradual tan is produced. If you are very fair-skinned, you will find it virtually impossible to go brown, however much you sunbathe, since your skin produces little pigment, and you are especially vulnerable to sunburn. Many suntanning preparations contain dyes that artificially color the skin. Others contain a colorless substance that turns the outer skin layer brown. This is not a true tan, because the pigment-producing cells have not been activated to produce melanin.

My father gets a cold sore when he sunbathes. What causes this?

Cold sores are a common viral infection of the skin. Most people are first infected in childhood, and the infection may pass unnoticed, but the virus remains latent in the cells of the skin. It may be reactivated by a stimulus such as sunlight, giving rise to a cold sore.

Why do I get pimples before a period?

This is very common in young women and is probably due to the fall in the hormone estrogen before a period.

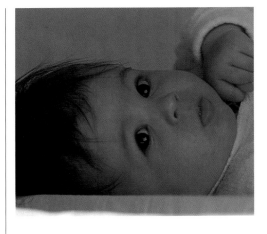

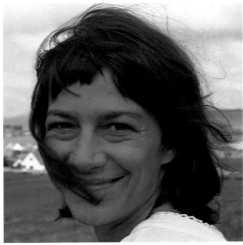

▲ ► How does a baby's smooth, firm skin become the wrinkled skin of an older person? The main reason for the aging of skin is damage to the elastic skin protein collagen by exposure to the ultraviolet component in sunlight. Those parts of the skin that are continuously protected from UVL by clothing show little deterioration. As cell growth slows down, an old skin cannot heal as quickly as a young one, and hair color and skin appearance fade.

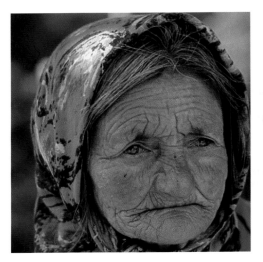

transformed into a material called keratin, which is finally shed as tiny, barely visible scales. It takes three to four weeks for a cell in the lowest layer to reach the surface.

This outer protective layer is firmly attached to an underlying layer called the dermis. Tiny, fingerlike bulges from the dermis fit into sockets in the epidermis, and this waviness at the junction of the two layers of skin gives rise to ridges, which are most obvious at the fingertips and give people their fingerprints. The dermis is made up from bundles of protein fibers called collagen and elastic fibers.

Glands and nerves

Embedded in the dermis are sweat, sebaceous, and apocrine glands; hair follicles; blood vessels; and nerves. The nerves penetrate the epidermis, but the blood vessels are confined to the dermis. The hairs and ducts from the glands pass through the epidermis to the surface of the skin.

Each sweat gland consists of a coiled tube of epidermal cells, which leads into the sweat duct to open out on the skin surface. The sweat glands are controlled by the nervous system and are stimulated to secrete by a release of emotion or by the body's need to lose heat (see Perspiration).

The sebaceous glands open into the hair follicles and are made up of specialized epidermal cells that produce grease or sebum to lubricate the hair shaft and surrounding skin. They are controlled by sex hormones and are most numerous on the head, face, chest, and back (see Sebaceous Glands).

The apocrine glands, a sexual characteristic, develop at puberty and are found in the armpits and breasts, and near the genitals. They are odor-producing and secrete a thick, milky substance.

There is a fine network of nerve endings in both the epidermis and the dermis, and they are particularly numerous at the fingertips. They transmit pleasurable sensations of warmth and touch, as well as cold, pressure, itching, and pain that may evoke protective reflexes (see Itches).

Hair and nails

Hair and nails are specialized forms of the protein keratin. Nails are produced by living cells, but the nail itself is dead and will not hurt or bleed if it is damaged. The visible part of the nail is called the nail body, and its shape is partly determined by genetic factors. The base of the nail,

STRUCTURE OF THE SKIN

The skin is made up from two layers of tissue: the epidermis and the dermis. Both layers contain nerve endings that transmit sensations. The sweat glands are vital in regulating the body's temperature; the sebaceous glands lubricate the skin and hair. The apocrine glands develop at puberty and are a sexual characteristic. The pigment-producing cells, called melanocytes, can cause freckles.

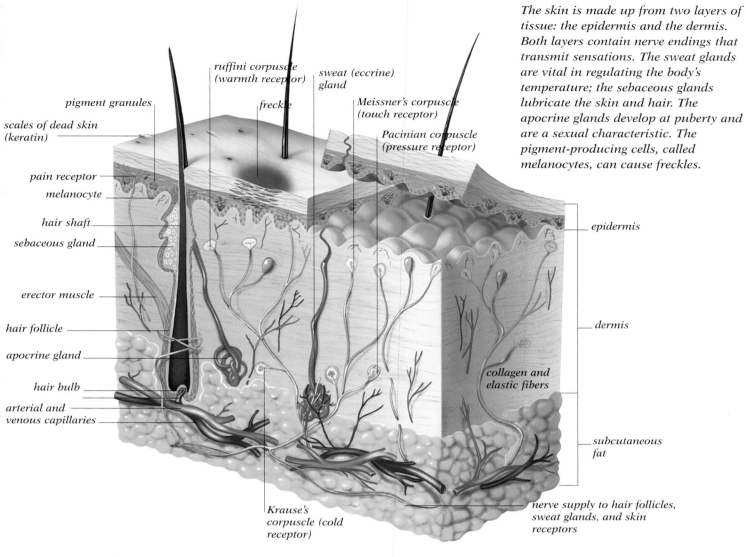

the root, is implanted in a groove in the skin. The cuticle overlaps the root, which is the site of active growth. As the living cells divide and move upward they become thick and tough, and when they die they form part of the nail itself (see Nails).

Hair is formed by cells in the hair follicles. There are two types: fine, downy hair, which is found over most of the body except the palms of the hands and soles of the feet; and thick, pigmented hair, which is present on the scalp, eyebrows, beard, and genital areas (see Genitals; Hair).

Hair grows in cycles, a long growing phase being followed by a short resting period. Hairs in the resting phase constitute up to 20 percent of the total 100,000 hairs on the scalp. The normal daily hair loss is between 20 and 100 hairs. Scalp hair grows about 0.3 inch (0.8 cm) per month. No single area is totally depleted at one time. The rapid growth of scalp hair makes it more susceptible to damage from disease, toxic drugs, and hormones.

The shape of our hair follicles is inherited, and this determines whether hair is straight or curly, together with the angle of the hair bulb in the shaft. If it lies straight, the hair will be straight; if bent, the hair will curl (see Heredity).

Skin color

Skin color is due to the black pigment melanin, which is produced by pigment cells in the lowest layer of the epidermis. There is the same number of pigment-producing cells in the skin of all races, but the amount of melanin produced varies. In dark-skinned people there is more melanin than in light-skinned people (see Melanin).

Other factors contributing to skin color are the blood in the blood vessels of the skin and the natural yellowish tinge of the skin tissue. The state of the blood within the blood vessels can greatly change skin color. Therefore, people become white with fear when small vessels close off, red with anger owing to an increased blood flow, and blue with cold because most of the oxygen in the blood moves out to the tissues when the blood flow slows down (see Oxygen).

Wound healing

All wounds heal by scar formation unless they are very superficial, such as a graze. Children heal faster than adults, but they also produce a larger quantity of scar tissue. However, scars in young people tend to resolve in time. As a general rule, dark pigmented skin heals with an excessive amount of scar tissue compared with light pigmented skin.

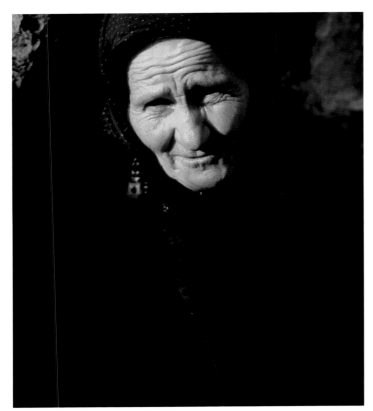

The healing process involves many changes. First the wound bleeds and becomes filled with a blood clot, which dries to form a scab. Blood vessels and fibrous tissue grow in from the cut surfaces of the wound, and the result is a scar that gradually becomes paler in color with time (see Scars; Wounds).

Skin conditions in children

Birthmarks are marks that are present on a baby's skin at birth, or that appear soon afterward. They include strawberry marks, moles, and port-wine stains. Many birthmarks do not require treatment and disappear of their own accord. Strawberry marks, for example, appear a few weeks after birth and grow rapidly for a while, but the majority disappear completely by the time a child is old enough to attend school (see Birthmarks).

Moles are not usually present at birth but develop during childhood, gradually increasing in size in adult life and sometimes disappearing late in life. Moles are formed from collections of the pigment-producing cells in the skin, and they may occasionally become malignant.

Babies and children have their own particular skin complaints. These include infant cradle cap, diaper rash, and chilblains. Cradle cap is a common condition that appears as a collection of scales and

◄▼ *The amount of melanin pigment in the skin is the major factor determining skin color, producing black and brown shades. Yellow tones are imparted by the pigment carotene.*

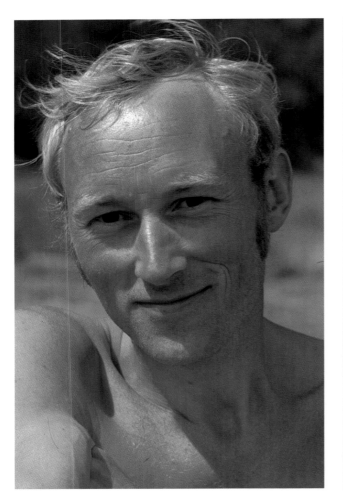

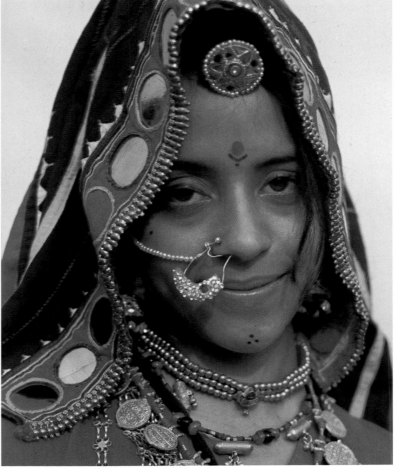

grease which stick together and adhere to the scalp. This can be removed by gentle shampooing after the scales have been softened with olive oil the night before.

Diaper rash is a red rash in the diaper area, which can spread to include the thighs and lower abdomen. It results from irritation produced by the bacterial decomposition of urine and feces. Because diaper rash is caused by the friction of a wet or soiled diaper, it is essential to change diapers frequently, leaving them off whenever possible, and avoiding the use of plastic pants. The skin should be washed with emulsifying lotions rather than soap, and water-repellent ointments that act as a barrier should be applied. Sometimes it is necessary to treat the rash with mild steroids containing antiinfective agents (see Diaper Rash; Steroids).

Eczema (atopic dermatitis) is a very common childhood problem resulting from an inherited state called atopy. This is a form of allergy to various substances such as house dust mite droppings, pollens, cat and dog hair, and some food ingredients. The skin is locally inflamed, scaly, and very itchy.

Chilblains are common in children who live in countries where the winters are cold. These sores occur on the toes, especially if tight-fitting shoes are worn, and on the fingers and ears. Sudden extreme changes in temperature should be avoided; although it is tempting to warm cold feet in front of the fire, this aggravates the condition. The affected area should be kept warm at all times.

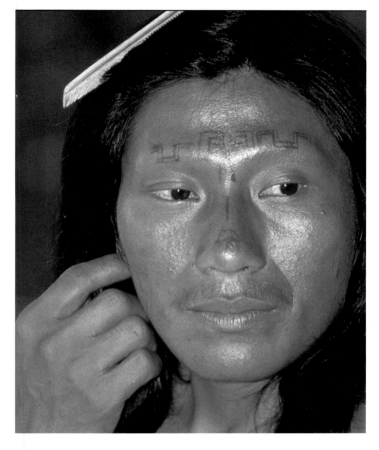

▼ ► *The pigment-producing cells are larger in dark-skinned people than fair-skinned races, but the number is constant. Dark-skinned people produce more melanin than fair people.*

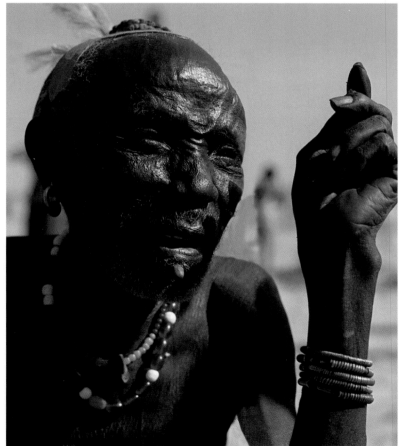

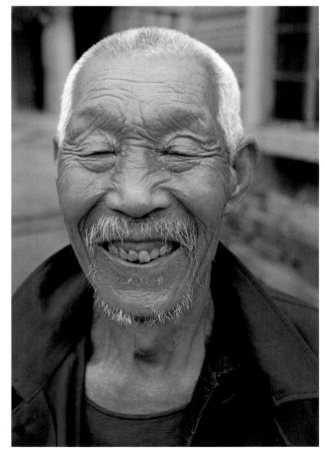

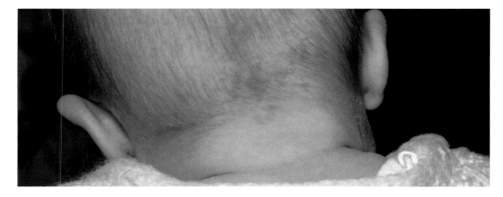

▲ *Many babies are born with superficial birthmarks. These do not need treatment and will disappear in time.*

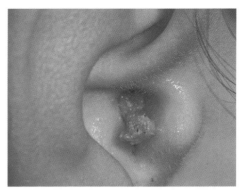

▲ *Warts are common in childhood, but simple treatments are usually effective.*

Infection of the skin often occurs in childhood because the skin's natural defenses have not yet been built up against bacteria, viruses, and fungi. Impetigo is a bacterial infection of the superficial layers of skin and is particularly likely to happen where skin is already damaged. It starts as a little red spot that enlarges and blisters to form a honey-colored crust . It is easily treated with antibiotics (see Impetigo).

Ringworm is caused by several kinds of fungi and gets its name from the ringed appearance of the rash. Sites most commonly affected are the scalp, groin, and feet. This skin complaint is rare in adults because of their greater immunity, and it is thought that the grease glands on the scalp may have some protective effect. Treatment is with antifungal preparations (see Ringworm).

Warts are the most common viral infection of the skin; most children catch warts as easily as they catch chicken pox. They tend to be found on the hands, knees, and soles of the feet, since the virus enters wherever the skin is broken. It lives in the outer layers of skin and causes very little damage, so a wart may pass unnoticed for months or even years. When the body becomes aware of the presence of the virus, it mobilizes its defenses and the wart may disappear as if by magic: hence the success of many wart charms and cures. Often the number of warts increases rapidly before they finally disappear (see Warts).

Since warts heal without leaving a scar, no treatment destructive enough to cause scarring should be used. Only simple wart paints should be applied, and the dead skin regularly pared away or frozen off. Treatment is usually successful, but may take two to three months before having an effect.

Skin conditions in adolescence

The hormonal changes that occur at puberty affect the skin chiefly by activating the grease-producing glands.

Sweating and blushing can be annoying problems for teenagers. Excessive sweating of

▲ *A malignant mole is characterized by itching, bleeding, or changes in color or size. Malignancies usually develop in adulthood, but if diagnosed early, a cure is possible.*

▼ *An allergic reaction is a common cause of dermatitis. For example, a person may find detergent irritating to the hands. Treatment would be to avoid contact by wearing rubber gloves.*

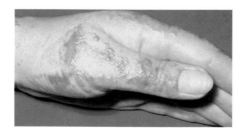

the armpits and hands, which is caused by emotion and heat, can be treated with aluminum chloride preparations applied locally. Blushing is not usually treated but tends to diminish as confidence increases.

Most teenagers develop a few acne spots that sometimes require medical attention. Acne appears sooner in girls than in boys because of the earlier onset of puberty. It usually resolves in the late teens and early twenties, but some people continue to need treatment up to the age of 30 or even 40. Acne is due to the excessive production of sebum or grease, which blocks the hair follicles. These then become infected with bacteria so that pimples and pustules form. Acne can and should be a successfully treated disease. Patients with mild acne require degreasing agents or keratolytics. Moderate or severe cases need oral antibiotics in addition to local treatment (see Antibiotics). Sunlight is usually beneficial because it dries up grease on the skin and helps to peel off the top layer.

Skin conditions in adults

As the skin ages there is a falling off in the production of natural emollients and it becomes dry. This drying process results in cracks in the skin, leaving it open to irritants at work or at home. Industrial dermatitis, where irritants are picked up in the workplace, is a more common cause of absence than any other industrial disease.

Dermatitis (skin inflammation) is thought to be mainly due to an external cause. Thus, those who use detergents at home may find their hands become irritated, while industrial dermatitis may be caused by many different substances, such as wet cement, chemicals, or fiberglass. Contact dermatitis is the result of an allergy to a substance, such as the nickel in jewelry. The cure is always avoidance of the cause.

Eczema is also common, giving rise to discomfort and disability at all ages. It presents different appearances at different stages, and may last from a few days to a lifetime. Initially there is reddening of the affected skin and itching, then pinhead swelling. Blisters then form, together with weeping and scaling. Eczema is often inherited, and is associated with asthma and hay fever. When all three occur in one person, the condition is known as atopic syndrome.

Caring for your skin

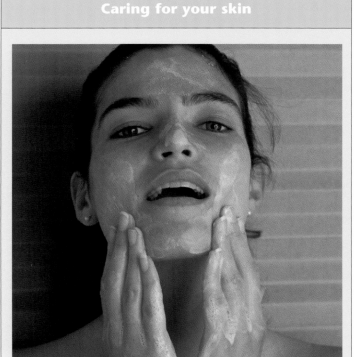

Skin care mainly consists of cleansing and moisturizing.

Cleansing creams are pure oil, and cleansing milks are oil in water. Both dissolve dirt and makeup without drying the skin too much. Cleansers that can be rinsed off are suited to all skin types.

Skin tonics refresh and stimulate the skin and should be applied after cleansing and before moisturizing. The simplest are distilled water and rosewater. Astringent lotions are more suited to oily skins because they help remove excess grease.

Moisturizers are creams with a low oil content. They slow down the rate of moisture evaporation from the skin.

Skin foods are heavy moisturizers with a high oil content; they are suitable for dry skins and nighttime use.

Cleanse oily skin with soap or a suitable cleanser and protect with a nonoily moisturizer.

Cleanse normal skin with mild soap or a liquid or cream cleanser. Use a moisturizer under makeup and at night.

Cleanse dry skin with a mild cleanser that can be rinsed away. Always use a moisturizer and night cream.

Eczema cannot be cured, but it can be controlled; it is not catching and does not leave scars. The skin of an eczema sufferer is more sensitive than normal; it is usually itchy and has a tendency to dryness. Steroids are the mainstay of treatment, and the weakest effective steroid is used. Irritants such as soap should be avoided, since they exacerbate the condition.

Skin allergies are often manifested in the development of urticaria or hives. The rash consists of white welts surrounded by reddened skin, which itches but does not last longer than a few hours. New welts may appear, however, so that the condition persists for days or weeks. The cause is often something that has been eaten—fruit or shellfish, for example—and some people are allergic to preservatives and synthetic dyes (see Hives).

The most common fungus infection of the skin is athlete's foot. The first signs are itching and peeling of the skin between the toes, which is often worse on one foot. Relapses are common in the summer, but the condition usually settles in cool weather and remedies are simple and effective (see Athlete's Foot).

Occasionally, a mole becomes malignant. Malignancy can occur in a mole that has been present for years, but if diagnosed early it can be removed and a cure is possible. Dubious-looking moles should always be removed. A malignant mole can arise at any age, though rarely in childhood (see Malignancy). The main cause is excessive exposure to sunlight. Malignant melanoma has become much more common in recent years mostly because of increased sunbathing. Only one mole in a million becomes a malignant melanoma (see Melanoma).

Hot flashes occur in women during menopause because of the hormonal changes at this time (see Menopause). Sometimes the flushing overstimulates the grease-producing glands to cause a condition called acne rosacea on the forehead, nose, cheeks, and chin. The sebaceous glands may enlarge to such an extent on the nose that it becomes bulbous and lumpy in appearance. The treatment of acne rosacea involves the avoidance of those things that aggravate flushing, particularly hot drinks. Prescribed oral antibiotics can also be very effective in severe cases (see Hot Flashes).

Skin conditions in older people

As the skin starts to age it not only dries out but also loses its former elasticity and does not heal so quickly or easily. The smallest wounds leave slight scars. Many older people also develop skin tags, sun-induced keratoses—grayish patches of skin—and seborrhoeic warts. These are brownish-black warty lesions that commonly appear on the body after the age of about 50. They are easily treated by freezing or by scraping off the lesion with a special surgical instrument.

The most common type of skin cancer is the rodent ulcer. These ulcers commonly occur in the United States, but are more generally found among fair-skinned people in sunny climates such as Australia. They usually occur on the face and neck and are slow-growing. These take the form of a hard, pearly-looking swelling, often with a dimple in the center and with a few fine red lines running over the edge. They do not spread remotely but can do much local deep damage (see Ulcers). Such ulcers are easily treated by local excision if they are small enough, or by radiotherapy. They are the least dangerous of cancers (see Cancer; Radiotherapy).

See also: **Acne and pimples; Allergies; Blisters; Blushing; Eczema; Glands; Hair and scalp disorders; Herpes; Rashes; Sunburn**

Sleep and sleep problems

Questions and Answers

Why can some people wake up and leap out of bed early, while I find getting up a real problem?

Patterns of sleeping and wakefulness are based on the way people's personal internal clocks work. Some people normally wake and get up early, whereas others go on feeling lively late into the night, but have trouble getting going in the morning—the night owls. Each group, in fact, has about the same amount of sleep, but it occurs at different times.

Why do babies spend so much time asleep?

Babies need to do a lot of growing in size and weight during their first few months of life, and sleep both conserves their energy and is a time when growth processes function best. Many people think that infants ought to spend virtually the whole of the 24 hours asleep, but this is not necessary. Other people think that most babies actually do spend almost all their time asleep. A few may, but if infants are observed around the clock, their total daily sleeping time turns out to be about 14 hours.

Are there aids to natural sleep?

Yes, several. A tired body and a quiet mind are important, so physical exercise, and mental relaxation in the form of reading, music, or television, can all help.

Is it possible to learn from tape-recorded information while asleep?

No. While you are asleep, your brain is not active enough to take in new material. The first half of the day, when your mind is rested, fresh, and uncluttered, is the best time to study and retain information, though of course many students study late at night.

People spend more of their lives asleep than in any other single activity. Difficulties in sleeping are very trying but can usually be overcome without recourse to sleeping pills, which should be regarded as only a last resort.

During a normal day people use up energy and tire themselves both physically and mentally. If people try to do without regular periods of rest they become exhausted. The most complete form of rest is sleep: for body and mind to be fresh and healthy, and to work efficiently, everyone needs to spend a part of every 24 hours sleeping. The body and mind do not stop working altogether during sleep; breathing continues and the heart continues to beat. Indeed, many parts of the body never rest; the eyelids flicker, people usually turn over several times and kick

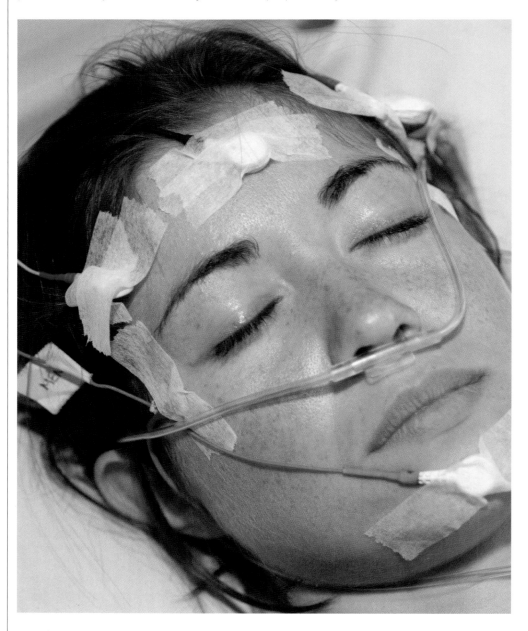

▲ *A woman is investigated for insomnia in a sleep observation laboratory.*

about, and some people talk and even walk about while they are asleep (see Sleepwalking). Even though vital processes, like respiration and the circulation of blood, continue while people are asleep, they do so at a much slower rate.

Brain activity

The sleep-wakefulness controls are located in the brain stem. Unless the brain cortex of the cerebral hemisphere, the thinking part of the brain, is activated by the brain stem, it is too torpid for conscious intellectual activity and it is said to be asleep. When someone is awake, the cerebral hemispheres are at a high pitch of activity, enabling the person to understand and respond to the things he or she sees and hears. The spinal cord is also highly tuned; it receives instructions from the brain to fire off carefully adjusted nerve messages that travel from the spinal cord cells along nerves to the muscles, which make the limbs move . Responsiveness in the cerebral cortex and in the spinal cord is brought about by electrical influences from the brain stem. When someone is awake the brain stem pours these currents along nerve channels and activates the cerebral hemispheres and spinal cord; the person then wakes up.

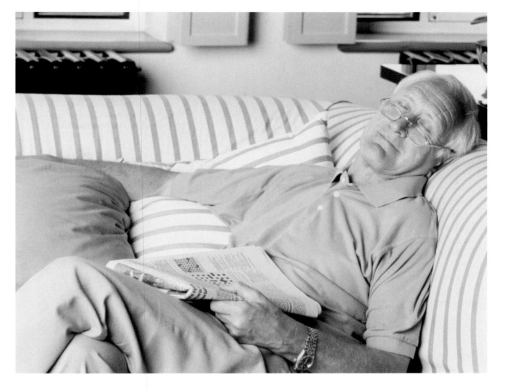

▲ *Relaxing in a comfortable, warm environment is enough to induce sleep.*

Several factors cause the brain stem sleep-wakefulness center to bring about wakefulness or sleep. What could be called a chemical clock induces sleep every 24 to 26 hours. The setting of the chemical clock is quite difficult to change, as becomes evident after a long flight to a country in a different time zone—France, for example, where clocks are set five to eight hours ahead of those in America. For the first week in a different time zone people sleep very late in the morning but feel wide awake when most inhabitants are going to bed. The sleep-wakefulness center is also much affected by lack of sleep. Of most importance are events taking place and their significance. No matter how sleepy a person feels, if a disturbance occurs, he or she will almost certainly wake up. The brain stem centers are stimulated by physical sensations, and especially by a change of sensation, but it is not only nerve messages from the body's sense organs that are stimulating during sleep. The sleep-wakefulness center also receives messages from the cortex of the cerebral hemispheres, so that any anxiety present in the mind bombards the brain stem with stimulating messages that induce wakefulness.

Another factor in keeping someone awake is new sensations. If the sights and sounds in the environment are monotonous and a person is immobile, there is nothing new to stimulate the brain stem, and sleep comes easily. A continuous rhythm, such as the clattering of train wheels, will add to the effect. A warm temperature and a comfortable chair will also help to bring about relaxation and sleep.

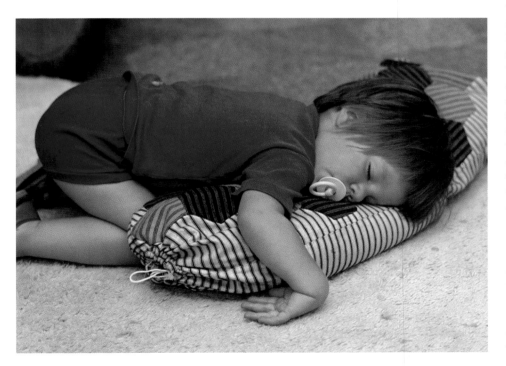

▲ *Young children sometimes resist daytime rests, but a comforter such as a special cushion or a pacifier can help a child relax enough to fall asleep.*

Questions and Answers

What is the best way to deal with children's nightmares?

Just as adults have nightmares, children have night terrors that they find frightening and distressing. The child may be temporarily disoriented during these episodes but usually the horror subsides and the child falls asleep again. However, the memory of the fear may linger, making the child fearful of going to bed or being left alone. Reprimanding or pleading with a child in this state is ineffectual; the child may feel rejected, and this will make the situation worse. The child finds nightly terror very real, so stay and read some stories, stroking the child's hair until he or she has fallen asleep. Keep a night-light on as well.

What are the dangers of taking sleeping pills on a regular basis?

It is undesirable to rely on drugs for a natural function like sleep. One problem is that some of the drugs have prolonged action and cause drowsiness the next day. It is often thought that since barbiturates were replaced by benzodiazepines, addiction to sleeping pills is less common. This is not so; drug dependence occurs with prolonged normal dosage of the newer drugs, and withdrawal symptoms—anxiety, agitation, irritability, and confusion—can be expected. Benzodiazepine drugs should be withdrawn gradually. Withdrawal symptoms will settle in three to four weeks depending on the personality of the patient.

Can prolonged sleeplessness make someone sick?

After about 60 hours without sleep a person will start seeing things that aren't there, or will fail to notice things that are. It becomes difficult to concentrate for more than a minute or so, and by 90 hours a person may suffer hallucinations. By 100 hours there may be signs of delirium. However, these symptoms persist only while sleep deprivation lasts.

HOW THE BRAIN CONTROLS SLEEP

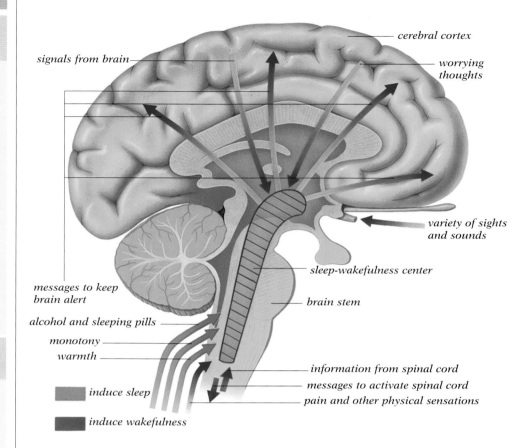

cerebral cortex

signals from brain

worrying thoughts

variety of sights and sounds

sleep-wakefulness center

messages to keep brain alert

brain stem

alcohol and sleeping pills

monotony

warmth

information from spinal cord

messages to activate spinal cord

pain and other physical sensations

induce sleep

induce wakefulness

▲ *The sleep-wakefulness center is located in the brain stem. Stimulated by information, including physical sensations, it passes messages to the cerebral cortex, which determines whether we fall asleep or stay awake. It also responds to signals from the cerebral cortex, so that a worrying thought can keep us awake. Equally, a quiet mind, warmth, certain drugs, and even monotony will induce sleep. The brain waves change as we become drowsy, sleep, and subsequently wake up refreshed.*

The brain stem centers are also affected by chemicals and drugs. Some, such as amphetamines, will prevent sleep whereas others, such as alcohol or sleeping pills, will have the opposite effect and cause drowsiness.

How much sleep do we need?

There are rare people who regularly devote less than three hours to sleep, and others who demand more than nine hours—everyone is different. The majority of adults average just under eight hours, while children sleep longer and older people sleep less than average.

Over a short period of time, a sleep debt can accumulate and, if someone is forced to make do with just a few hours of sleep for a period of days or weeks, it will take more than an average eight hours at the weekend or on vacation to compensate. Although at times someone may manage to keep going on a reduced sleep ration, he or she probably does not feel really well and almost certainly are not as efficient, nor so attentive to detail in daily tasks.

Dreaming

No one can do without sleep; and everyone needs two different kinds of sleep. A definite pattern of events occurs during prolonged sleep; there will be increased restlessness, changes in the electrical brain waves, and spells of rapid eye movement which happen about every one and a half hours, and which last for 20 minutes each time. If people are deliberately woken during the

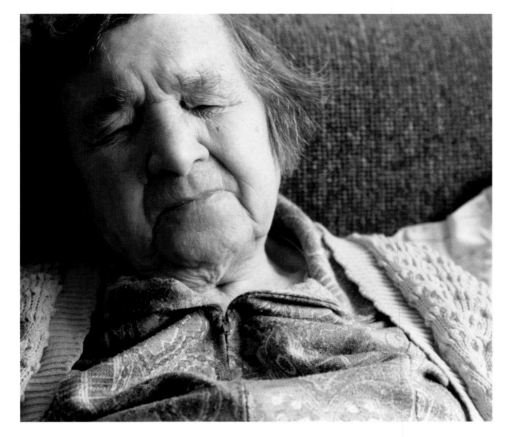

▲ *Elderly people like this woman often find it very easy to slip into a light sleep or doze, and can awake from it just as easily.*

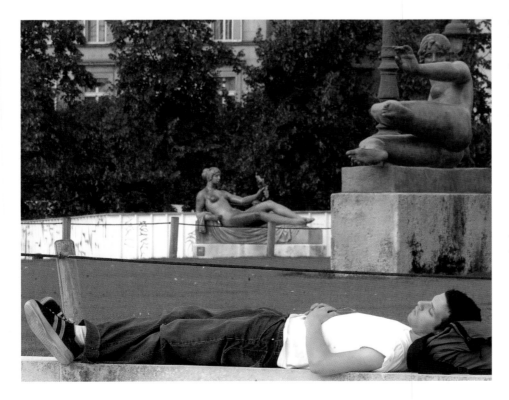

▲ *After eating or drinking, fresh air and sunshine can induce relaxation and then sleep—even on a rather uncomfortable bed.*

rapid eye movement periods, they usually say they have just been dreaming (see Rapid Eye Movement Sleep). If woken at other times they usually say they have not been dreaming and, indeed, have apparently forgotten the dream that presumably accompanied the previous rapid eye movement period. They may say they had been reviewing the day's events; not colorful, adventurous dreaming, but nevertheless not a total absence of mental life. Mental activity therefore seems to continue, often at a low ebb, throughout the whole period of sleep, although most people scarcely remember it.

REM sleep

The rapid eye movement phase of sleep is known as REM, or paradoxical, sleep. In these phases the electrical brain waves are faster than in the orthodox, non-rapid eye movement or NREM phases. The heart rate, breathing, and blood pressure undergo rapid fluctuations during paradoxical sleep, especially at the time of a sudden flurry of eye movements. Most bodily muscles are completely relaxed, the usual reflexes are absent, in men the penis is often erect, the blood flows more rapidly through the brain, and less flows through the muscles. At these times there is dreaming.

Mental activity during REM sleep is concerned with sorting out and making sense of disconnected items of memorized material. In the orthodox phase of sleep into which we always pass for an hour or so before moving into the paradoxical phase, brain waves are large and slow. Electrical activity of most individual brain cells is reduced, but at this time growth hormone is poured into the blood.

Adults do not grow taller, but growth, repair, and the renewal of many tissues, such as skin, liver, or blood-forming cells in the bone marrow, must continue. At some unknown signal from the chemical clock, these cells start to divide as the usual time for sleep approaches. Then, during the orthodox sleep phase, growth hormone is released. It is this hormone that helps the newly divided cells of the body to grow into complete new cells (see Hormones).

Adults do not grow new brain cells, although they do still need to renew the cells' constituents. It seems that the paradoxical phase of sleep, with plenty of blood flowing through the brain, is a time when this renewal is most active. When the brain is actually growing, at the time of birth, the paradoxical phase takes up twice the proportion of sleep it does a few months later, when brain growth has slowed down.

Babies and sleep

A favorite remark of many child care experts is that young babies do not suffer from sleep problems—but their parents do. In general a baby will sleep when, and for as long as, it needs. Problems arise only when a baby does not seem to need the amount of sleep that its parents think appropriate. At this stage a baby cannot inhibit sleep or wake up on purpose. It makes no difference to a baby if it sleeps all day and plays all night, but its parents cannot afford to follow a similar pattern. A baby has to be gradually persuaded to accept the usual daily rhythm of sleeping at night. Most people surface several times in the night, and babies are no exception. If each of a baby's brief awakenings brings a hovering, anxious parent to its side, a baby will not ignore an opportunity for sociability. An overattentive mother can prevent her baby from learning to settle back to sleep by itself, and therefore reinforces a pattern of disturbed sleep.

While slight rustlings and grumbles are probably best ignored, loud crying demands prompt attention. Toward the second year of life, nightmares begin to be common, although in a child not yet talking we cannot know much about such night fears. A child wakes suddenly, usually with a scream, and gives every appearance of being terrified. Usually all that is needed is a reassuring hug to settle the child back to sleep.

Problems in persuading a child to fall asleep in the first place can also arise around this time. Often it seems that what a baby resents is not sleep itself but the separation from its mother that sleep entails. Parents have to try to get a child to understand that there is no need to cry because there is no danger of being abandoned, and that there is no point in crying because it is now time to sleep. Visiting a child every five minutes or so while he or she continues to fuss, but staying just long enough to smile and repeat good night can often help a child to settle. If left alone to cry, a child will eventually exhaust itself and fall asleep, but he or she may be quicker to make a fuss the following night.

Insomnia

Difficulties in sleeping are a common and disturbing adult complaint. Insomnia (see Insomnia) may manifest itself as difficulty in getting to sleep, interrupted sleep, or waking too early. Worry, tension, and depression are by far the most common causes, but pain, uncomfortable surroundings, fever, breathing difficulties on lying down (orthopnea), a need to pass urine frequently, and dyspepsia that is worse on lying down—for example, if someone has a hiatus hernia—may also give rise to insomnia.

Persistent sleeplessness soon begins to cause daytime problems such as drowsiness, lack of concentration, and irritability. There are many ways people can help themselves if they suffer from

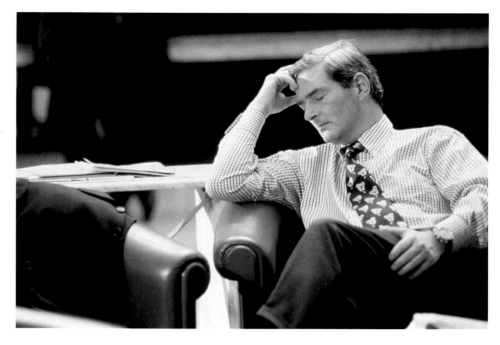

▲ *Some people are able to function after only three hours of sleep a night. Many people can catnap during their working day and wake completely refreshed.*

sleeplessness. It is important to make sure that no unresolved tensions are left over from the day, because tension and stress are common causes of sleep problems. If possible, family arguments should be settled before it is time to sleep. An exercise that can help is for someone, once in bed, to go over all the events of the day from the time of awakening. Events happen so fast during the day that the mind cannot digest them properly, and this can disturb sleep.

The environment for sleeping is important. Quietness, warmth, and a firm mattress are good investments. Adequate physical fatigue can be important (see Fatigue); it helps if the body is tired as well as the mind. If a person does not get much exercise at work, a late-night walk can be a successful way of dealing with insomnia. When someone is trying to resolve a problem in the mind that prevents relaxation and sleep, spending half an hour reading a good book or listening to music is much less stressful, and more effective, than being wakeful in bed.

Any difficulty in sleeping that goes on for more than two weeks should be referred to a doctor. By this time the cause needs to be identified and treated. Sleeping pills and tranquilizers (see Tranquilizers) should be regarded as a last resort; they are addictive and have the effect of changing someone into a person who is less alert, less aware, and less alive. However, there are times of exceptional stress and upset in most people's lives when they may have to resort to pills or tranquilizers for short periods. If such drugs are prescribed, a doctor's advice must be followed on how to take them, but a recommended way is to take an adequate dose about half an hour before bedtime in order to ensure sleep.

This regimen should be followed for three, four, or five nights; then the dose should be halved on the succeeding three nights; after that, a person should take the pills only if he or she is still feeling restless an hour after going to bed.

See also: Brain; Spinal cord

Sleepwalking

Questions and Answers

Is the act of sleepwalking at all dangerous?

Sleepwalkers often bump into things, but in general they seem to avoid large obstacles. However, there have been reports of sleepwalkers falling down stairs and even from open windows. This is why every effort should be made to prevent a sleepwalker in the family from injuring him- or herself.

Do more men walk in their sleep than women?

No. This is an old theory, but research carried out to investigate the incidence of sleepwalking in various populations discovered no gender bias.

Can somnambulism be inherited?

Sleep disturbances in general, and sleepwalking in particular, seem to run in families. However, it should be remembered that it is no proof of inheritance that a behavior runs in a family, even when many members of the family are apparently affected. In the case of sleepwalking, a genetic, rather than an environmental cause, is unlikely.

Can sleepwalking be cured?

It is usually outgrown, but if it continues to occur frequently, a doctor may prescribe drugs that suppress the deeper phases of sleep. Because treatment can be unpredictable, many doctors prefer to refer a persistent sleepwalker to a psychiatrist.

Is it dangerous to wake a sleepwalker suddenly?

No, but being woken up suddenly can be confusing or, in the case of children, even terrifying.

Sleepwalking usually occurs in children between the ages of six and 12. The occasional sleepwalking episode is a normal occurrence, especially in children, and most children will outgrow the problem.

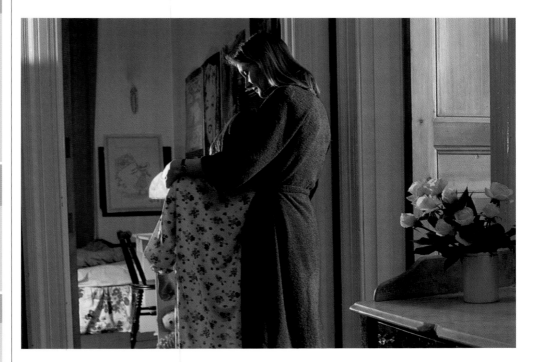

▲ *Never wake a child found sleepwalking, since this may cause confusion and fear; rather, gently lead him or her back to bed. In time the child should outgrow the habit.*

Sleepwalking, a condition known as somnambulism, is a disorder that occurs most commonly in children, but sometimes also in adults. It is thought to affect about 2 percent of the population.

It was once believed that sleepwalking involved the physical acting out of a dream, and that it took place during periods of shallow sleep. However, experiments have revealed that sleepers walk during the deepest phases of sleep. Most episodes last only a few minutes (see Dreaming).

Sleepwalkers observed in laboratories walk with open, yet expressionless, eyes, giving them a blank or dazed look. Some do no more than sit up in bed and lie down again, while others walk around aimlessly, in a rigid, robotlike fashion. They often rub some object repetitively. Most walkers eventually go back to bed of their own accord, and all may eventually be led back without difficulty. In every case, when they wake up they remember nothing about the incident.

The belief that this disorder indicates deep psychological problems is an old one. In the case of children, if it happens only occasionally, the claim that sleepwalking is due to psychological problems is usually unfounded; sleepwalking is a perfectly normal activity. However, the disorder in adults is sometimes an indication of emotional disturbance. The causes are not yet fully understood; it has been suggested that there may be a fault with the mechanism of waking up.

Children normally grow out of the habit of sleepwalking, and sleepwalkers seldom harm themselves, but precautions are advisable. Doors and windows should be locked; potentially dangerous objects such as electric appliances and sharp items should be removed from the sleepwalker's room. When someone walks in his or her sleep, the walker should be led back to bed without being awakened; this could cause disorientation or terror.

See also: Sleep and sleep problems

Slipped disk

Questions and Answers

Does sleeping with a board under the mattress help to prevent a slipped disk?

No, it won't prevent a slipped disk from occurring. Many people with back problems find that a firm mattress helps their back because it is more comfortable. A soft mattress can sag in the middle so that lying on the bed bends the back. This is an uncomfortable position; you would not like to walk about all day with a bent back. Putting a hard board under a soft mattress is an inexpensive and effective way of making a bed more comfortable.

Are women more prone to slipped disks than men?

No. Two to three times as many men as women suffer from a slipped disk. The reasons for this are not clear, and, contrary to popular belief, heavy physical work is not associated with a greater risk of a slipped disk. However, a slipped disk is obviously more troublesome to a heavy manual worker than to someone with a sedentary lifestyle. Pregnant women are much more likely to develop a slipped disk. The increase in weight puts an additional strain on the back. Hormones secreted during pregnancy may also cause a general softening of the ligaments and the muscles.

What causes a slipped disk to rupture and what happens?

All slipped disks are in fact ruptured disks. The disk is made of a tough outer ring and a soft inner core. A slipped disk occurs when the tough outer ring weakens, so the soft inner material bulges out and presses on the nerves of the spinal cord. If the outer ring cracks, the inner material can escape into the area of the spinal cord.

A slipped, or prolapsed, disk can cause a lot of pain and temporarily restrict normal movement. In a large majority of cases, however, letting nature take its course results in a patient's full recovery.

CLASSIC SLIPPED DISK

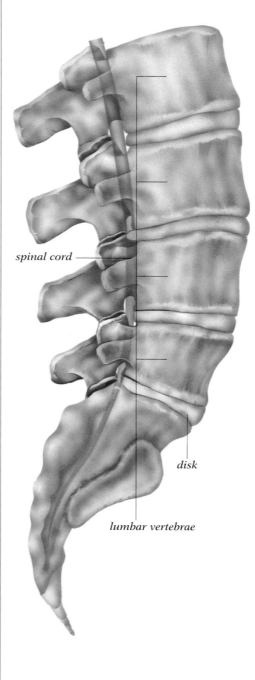

spinal cord

disk

lumbar vertebrae

▲ *A slipped disk usually occurs in the lower spine (the lumbar region).*

Back problems are an extremely common cause of pain and suffering, and many days of work are lost in the United States through backache. There are many causes of back problems, of which a slipped disk is only one of a range of possibilities (see Back and Backache). Although many cases of backache improve with time, medical treatment should be sought if the pain is persistent or particularly severe.

What is a slipped disk?

The disks are pads of tissue situated between each of the vertebrae that make up the spinal column. Each disk consists of a tough, fibrous outer ring called the annulus fibrosus and a softer, jellylike inner layer called the nucleus pulposus. The function of the disk is to act as both a strong connection between the vertebrae and a cushion to absorb weight on the spinal column.

A slipped disk does not really slip; the tough outer fibrous ring (annulus) cracks open and the softer inner layer protrudes

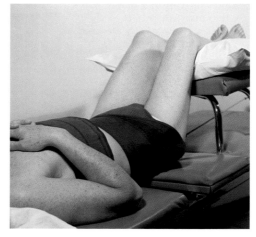

▲ *Over 90 percent of people with a slipped disk recover by resting in bed for between three days and three weeks. If the symptoms persist, patients may have to spend time in the hospital with their legs supported in such a way that pressure on the nerves can be relieved.*

(prolapses) through the crack, like toothpaste coming out through a crack in a toothpaste tube. For this reason doctors prefer to speak of a disk prolapse rather than a slipped disk.

The nucleus of a disk is softest and most jellylike during childhood. Over the years the nucleus gradually dries out so that by middle age it has a consistency similar to crabmeat. As someone gets older, the nucleus becomes even firmer. In elderly people the disk is mainly a section of scar tissue; this accounts for the fact that old people lose height. Disk protrusion occurs less frequently as people get older; it is a disorder affecting young adults and people in early middle-age. Disk protrusion occurs where the outer layer of the disk is weakest; that is, just in front of the nerve roots, which emerge from the spinal cord at each vertebral level. There is very little free space within the spinal canal, and the protruding disk material presses on the nerve root at that level and causes the painful symptoms of a slipped disk (see Spinal Cord).

The area of the spine most likely to be affected is the lowermost part of the back. Here the greatest strains occur, and it is not surprising that most disks that fail are at this level. However, it is possible for disks to prolapse at any level along the length of the spinal column—in the back or the neck.

Causes

The disk begins to prolapse when a crack develops in its tough outer ring. This is usually the effect of wear and tear in the back as a result of normal aging. One particularly heavy or awkward lift, a fall, or even a sudden cough or sneeze may force some of the soft disk nucleus to prolapse, leading to sudden symptoms.

Symptoms

When a prolapsing disk presses on a nerve root, symptoms occur both in the back and in the area that the nerve root supplies. For example, a slipped disk in the lower back can cause pain in the legs.

Symptoms in the back can include severe backache. Often the sufferer will not be able to localize the pain with any accuracy. He or she may also develop painful spasms in the muscles that lie along each side of the spine, particularly in the early stages. The patient will feel more pain when moving about and some relief when lying flat. Coughing or sneezing can cause the prolapsing disk material to bulge out suddenly, causing a sharp pain in the back or legs. In addition there may be a curvature of the spine—the patient unconsciously leans away from the side of the disk prolapse to try to relieve the pressure from the nerve root that is involved.

If the pressure on the nerve root is not too severe, the nerve will continue to work but will be painful. The brain cannot tell that the painful pressure is coming from the area of the disk, but instead interprets the information as pain originating in the nerve end. In a lower-back disk protrusion the sciatic nerve can be irritated, and the individual may feel pain in the thigh, calf, ankle, or foot. This pain can shoot down a leg and is then called sciatica.

More severe pressure on the nerve root may cause the nerve to stop functioning altogether. Areas of skin that the nerve supplies will become numb, so that a light touch or even a pinprick cannot be felt. Muscles supplied by the nerve will become weak or even completely paralyzed. Reflexes such as the knee-jerk reflex may disappear. If only one nerve root is involved this is not too serious, because each nerve supplies only a small area of skin, or a limited number of muscles. If the nerves to the bladder or genitals are affected, however, their function can be permanently lost. Urgent medical attention is needed to relieve the pressure on these nerves.

Treatment

Well over 90 percent of people with acute disk protrusions get better simply by resting in bed. The soft inner disk material tends to dry up and shrink once it has prolapsed, thus relieving the pressure on the nerve root. The main form of treatment is rest. Once the doctor has examined the individual and confirmed that there is a straightforward disk prolapse, he or she will advise the patient to rest as much as possible by lying flat in bed. In the horizontal position the pressure within the disk (acting in order to force out the soft inner material) is minimal. In the standing position this pressure is higher, and when the back is bent—for example, when a person is sitting or bending over—the pressure is much higher. A soft bed also bends the back, so it is best to put boards under the mattress or even to put the mattress on the floor.

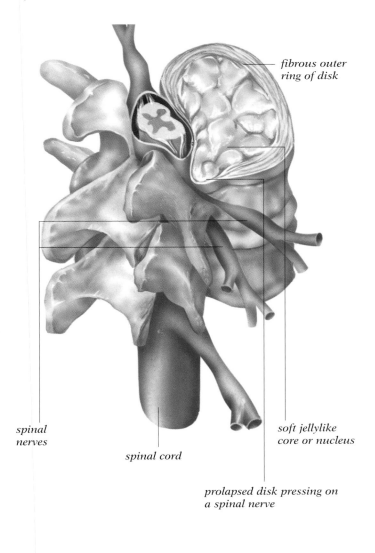

fibrous outer ring of disk

spinal nerves

spinal cord

soft jellylike core or nucleus

prolapsed disk pressing on a spinal nerve

▲ A slipped disk most frequently occurs in the lower spine. The tough outer layer of the disk weakens, allowing the soft inner core, or nucleus, to bulge out, causing pain and muscle weakness. When the protrusion presses on a nearby spinal nerve, feeling may be lost in the lower part of the body.

Questions and Answers

I strained my back when lifting a heavy chair. Does this mean I had a slipped disk?

The back consists of a series of bones, ligaments, disks, and muscles. Injury to any of these may occur in lifting heavy objects incorrectly. This can cause acute pain in the back, which may extend to the legs. Get your doctor to establish if the pain was caused by a slipped disk.

Is it possible to cure a slipped disk by surgery?

Yes. Although 90 percent of people suffering from a slipped disk recover within two months, a small number of patients will need surgery. Such operations are used for patients whose slipped disk has shown up clearly on a special X ray and who have not responded to other treatment. Occasionally a patient with a severe slipped disk, which is pressing on the nerves to the bladder, will need emergency treatment to relieve the pressure. Surgery for slipped disks is successful in the vast majority of cases. Around 85 percent of patients recover from their back pain, or else their condition is greatly improved.

My doctor thinks that I may have a slipped disk, and she is sending me to the hospital to have a spinal X ray. Can you tell me what will happen?

The X ray your doctor has recommended is called a myelogram. A dye is injected into the membranes surrounding the nerves in the spinal cord. This dye is opaque to X rays. If you have a slipped disk, the disk will protrude and this will show up as an indentation in the column of dye. If an emerging nerve is not outlined by the dye, this shows that the nerve has been compressed.

An operation, called a laminectomy, may then be performed to push aside the spinal cord and nerve roots in order to remove the disk material.

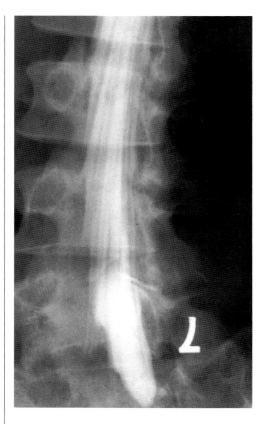

▲ *A special X ray, a myelogram (above), is used to diagnose a slipped disk.*

Painkilling drugs are of help in alleviating the pain in acute disk prolapse, although they will probably not take it away altogether (see Painkillers). Drugs that relax the muscles, such as diazepam (Valium), help to settle painful muscle spasm.

Most patients will get better if they rest in bed for up to three weeks. Great patience is needed—there is no way that nature's healing processes can be speeded up. Getting up too soon will often result in a relapse.

Patients who fail to make a recovery after a proper course of bed rest may require further treatment. This may entail a period of hospitalization, perhaps with traction to the legs to help relieve the pain.

If this fails, a special X ray may be necessary. X rays show only the bones of the spine—the disk itself shows only as a space between the bones. This space is altered in an acute disk prolapse. The special X ray is called a myelogram or radiculogram. A dye which shows up on X rays is injected into the space just outside the spinal canal; if the disk has in fact prolapsed, it will show as an indentation in the column of dye. A magnetic resonance scan may also be useful to determine whether the disk has prolapsed (see Diagnostic Imaging; Scans; X Rays).

BACK STRAIN AND PRESSURE

The vertebrae in the small of the back (lumbar vertebrae) take most strain. This chart assumes that when you are standing the pressure on your lumbar vertebrae is normal, or 1.00. Pressure is reduced to 0.25, or a quarter, when you are lying flat, but increases threefold if you are sitting while holding weights.

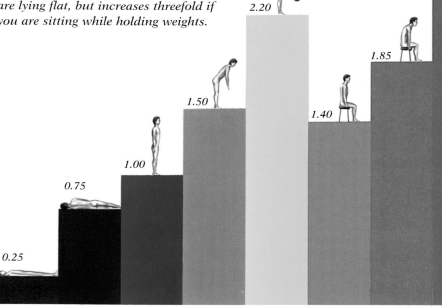

2.75

2.20

1.85

1.50

1.40

1.00

0.75

0.25

Surgery to remove prolapsed disk material may be necessary if bed rest fails to improve the symptoms, if there are signs of rapidly worsening function of nerve roots, or if the nerves to the bladder or the genitals are involved.

The operation (a laminectomy) involves making a small opening in the bones surrounding the spinal cord and gently pushing them aside, along with the nerve roots, to remove the disk material. Patients can usually become mobile within two weeks of this surgery.

Surgery for prolapsed disk has developed a bad reputation among the public, probably because in the past diagnosis was not always accurate and careful selection of those patients most likely to benefit from surgery was not always undertaken. With modern methods the success rate of surgery is high.

Many people suffering from disk prolapse receive other forms of treatment such as physical therapy and manipulation. Physical therapy may consist of heat treatment, which temporarily lessens the pain, and traction exercises. Traction helps to relieve pain by decreasing muscle spasm. Exercises help to strengthen the muscles of the back and stomach so that they can take strain off the bones and joints in the spine (see Physical Therapy).

Manipulation is practiced by many physical therapists, some doctors, and all osteopaths (see Manipulation; Osteopathy). The aim is to move the protruding disk material away from its point of contact with the nerve root and to free the nerve from any inflammation. There is no evidence to show that the soft prolapsing disk material can actually be returned to the firm outer casing—this would be like trying to put toothpaste back into its tube—but enough movement to take some pressure off the nerve root may be achieved. Manipulation is probably more useful in other types of back disorders, although some individuals receive excellent results for prolapsed disk.

Another useful treatment is to administer an epidural injection. A quantity of local anesthesia mixed with steroids is injected into the space just outside the spinal canal, so that it reaches the nerve roots where they emerge from the spinal cord. This is often combined with manipulation of the legs in order to move the sciatic nerve and to break down any small pieces of scar tissue that have formed around the nerve roots. This treatment is used when sciatica persists after the other signs of an acute disk prolapse have settled. It often gives immediate relief from pain.

Other aids

Back supports, corsets, and plaster jackets are used by some doctors to prevent patients from bending their backs during the recovery period after a disk prolapse. Long-term use of a corset tends to weaken the back muscles so that the patient becomes uncomfortable when not wearing the support.

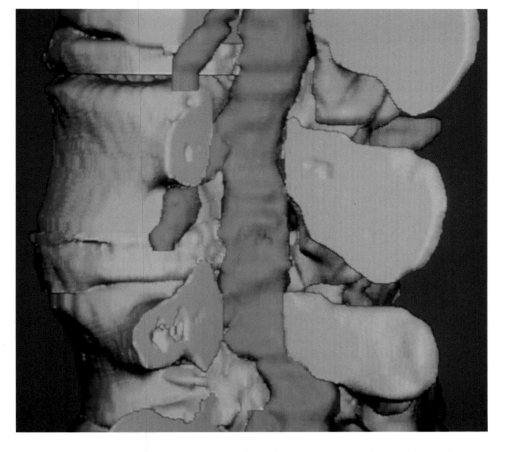

▲ *A CT scan clearly shows a slipped disk (yellow; lower center) pressing against the spinal cord (dark blue). The vertebrae (light blue) have been revealed in cross section by computer image manipulation.*

Prevention

People who have suffered from a disk prolapse and those who are at risk of a prolapse because of their occupation must learn to look after their backs. Proper lifting procedures such as keeping the back straight, bending at the knees rather than bending the back when picking things up from the floor, and avoiding lifting too much weight are important. It is also vital to keep body weight under control. Extra weight puts additional strain on the back. Regular exercise will increase the efficiency of the back muscles. Swimming is a particularly beneficial form of exercise, since the effects of gravity are eliminated and the back is not placed under undue strain.

Outlook

Some individuals fail to make a full recovery even after they have received adequate treatment. It may be necessary for people in strenuous occupations to find a less demanding job. The sufferer may have to change to a less active lifestyle and also recognize factors that affect the back. The sympathetic understanding of employers, relatives, and friends is important for such people.

The large majority of people who suffer from disk prolapse recover completely and are able to return to their previous activities. The recovery process may take several months, but patience is usually rewarded with a good result.

See also: **Exercise; Sciatica**

Smallpox

This disease was once the scourge of humankind. It ravaged populations and left disfiguring scars on survivors' faces. Smallpox was eradicated in 1979, but anxiety over its possible use as a terrorist weapon continues.

Questions and Answers

Is it still necessary to have a smallpox vaccination before visiting another country?

No, it is not necessary. The disease is now thought to have been eradicated from all parts of the world.

Could a person have caught smallpox when he or she was vaccinated?

Yes, this might have happened, and the illness could have been severe. However, people were much less likely to have died from the illness if they had been vaccinated. Doctors and nurses who worked in isolation hospitals were vaccinated and they still sometimes got a mild form of pneumonia, which was the way the disease expressed itself in an immunized person.

Is it true that pregnant women can't have a smallpox vaccination?

Yes. The vaccinia virus that gives immunity against smallpox crosses over the placenta and may infect the baby, inducing a miscarriage. Smallpox was a devastating disease in pregnancy. The baby was likely to become infected, and therefore abort. The disease in the mother was often more severe than normal.

I remember that when I was a child I could not have a smallpox vaccination. Why was this?

Probably you suffered from eczema. Normally the vaccination produced a single spot on the arm. However, people with eczema, especially children, could develop eczema all over their bodies, and this was sometimes fatal. Thus children with eczema were not vaccinated against smallpox, even when there was a chance of catching the disease.

▲ *This document, dated December 9, 1979, declares the world officially free from smallpox. Even as late as 1967 smallpox was endemic in large areas of the world, but the disease was finally cornered in eastern Africa and eradicated.*

Smallpox was once the most common of the dangerous, fatal virus diseases. However, the World Health Organization declared the world free from the disease in 1979. This is one of the most remarkable successes of preventive medicine that the world has yet seen. However, before this, the disease was widespread, and many people are still marked by the scars left by the smallpox spots.

Causes

Two strains of the virus, called variola major and variola minor, caused smallpox. As the names suggest, one strain caused a less serious disease than the other, although infection with the variola minor strain was still extremely serious, sometimes even fatal.

One of the reasons why the virus was so successful was that it was able to survive easily outside the human body. It could withstand temperatures of -94°F (-70°C), and was stable at up to 131°F (55°C). Therefore the virus could survive in crusts of skin for months at room temperature, especially since it could easily resist the effect of drying.

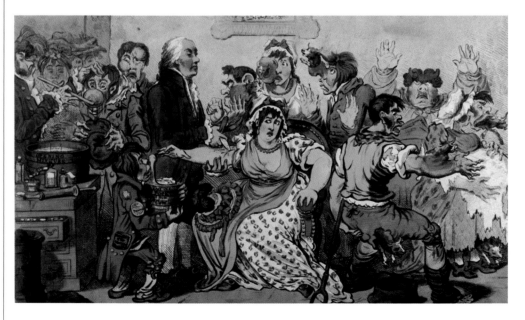

▲ *Public reaction to Jenner's great 18th-century breakthrough, the discovery that cowpox vaccination protected against smallpox, was lampooned by the cartoonist James Gillray.*

REPORTED CASES OF SMALLPOX IN 1967

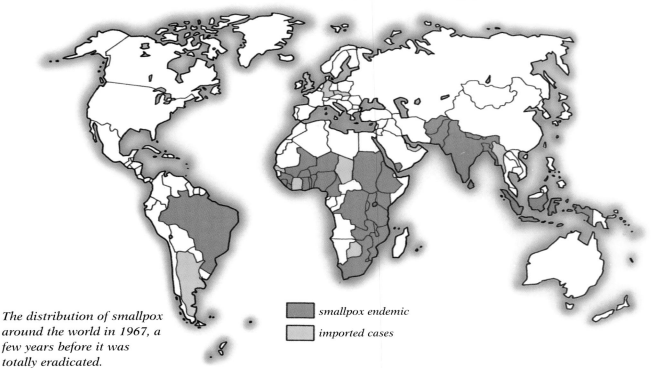

The distribution of smallpox around the world in 1967, a few years before it was totally eradicated.

smallpox endemic

imported cases

Like so many virus infections, the disease was spread by airborne liquid droplets. The virus was shed into the saliva from the circulating blood and then breathed out, to be inhaled by the next human contact. In epidemics, each infected person passed the disease on to about five other people, usually those in very close contact. The disease had a fixed incubation period of about 12 days; therefore, epidemics would tend to build up, with new waves of cases occurring every two weeks or so (see Viruses).

Symptoms

During the incubation period the disease spread from the nose and throat and into the lymphatic system. The prodromal phase of the illness followed: the interval between the first symptoms and the appearance of the raised spots. It was in this stage that the disease made people feel very sick. There was fever, with aching muscles and limbs; and the prodromal rash, which was a simple outcrop of spots, surrounded by bleeding in very severe cases. This rash progressed to raised spots and then fluid-filled pox spots known as vesicles. After three or four days, the smallpox vesicles became cloudy and were then called pustules. Finally, after about nine days the rash formed a hard crust. Crusted pustules would then heal, but they could leave serious scars.

Dangers and treatment

There were various ways of predicting the severity of smallpox. In variola major, copious bleeding around the rash signaled a very high risk of death—more than 95 percent. A very deep, flat rash could mean mortality of over 80 percent. Less severe forms of the disease could still show mortality of 30 percent in unvaccinated people, with the severity of the disease being proportional to the extent of the rash (see Rashes).

Even vaccinated people could contract variola major, albeit a much milder form, and the mortality rate was still about 1 percent. Variola minor was a separate strain of the virus, and the overall mortality rate was about 1 percent of cases. However, in all cases and types of smallpox, the cause of death was due not to any complications of the disease, but to the virulent attack of the virus itself on the body tissues. In the severe form of variola major, when bleeding around the pox spots occurred, death was caused about 48 hours after the onset by bleeding into internal organs. More often, however,

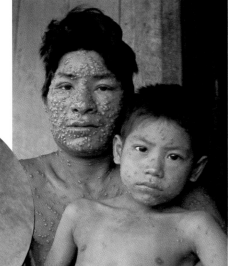

◄▲ This electron microscope picture shows the characteristic brick shape of the variola virus that caused smallpox. Spread by droplet infection, it brought fever, aching muscles, and a disfiguring rash (above).

Could you catch smallpox just by traveling on the same bus or airplane as someone suffering from the disease?

Smallpox was one of the most infectious diseases. However, as with any other similar disease you would have been most likely to catch it from someone in your immediate family. The last case in Britain happened as a result of a laboratory accident. The virus, kept in the laboratory for research purposes, spread through the ventilating system to infect a worker on the floor above. The person died, and the incident demonstrated all too clearly that close personal contact was not always required for the disease to be transmitted.

Did everyone with smallpox die from the disease?

There were two strains of smallpox that produced a rather similar disease. One of them, called variola major, produced a disease that had an overall mortality of about 40 percent in people who had not been vaccinated. Variola minor, the other form, produced a similar disease that was less severe and was rarely fatal.

After recovery from smallpox, was there any permanent damage?

As with chicken pox, the actual rash could leave severe scarring, and smallpox had a tendency to affect the face. In a few cases the eyes were involved and the smallpox could then scar the cornea, causing blindness.

Could smallpox be caught from animals?

No, and this was largely why it was possible to eradicate the disease. Other serious diseases can live in animals, so that humans can get reinfected. Lassa fever, for example, is carried by rats, and malaria is carried by mosquitoes, so these diseases are difficult to eradicate completely.

ERADICATION OF SMALLPOX

▼ *Outbreaks of smallpox occurred in waves, the early 1950s and the mid-1960s being particularly bad. In 1967 the policy of global eradication was intensified. Aided by worldwide cooperation, rapid diagnosis, isolation, and mass vaccination, the disease was finally eradicated in 1979 and is now a thing of the past.*

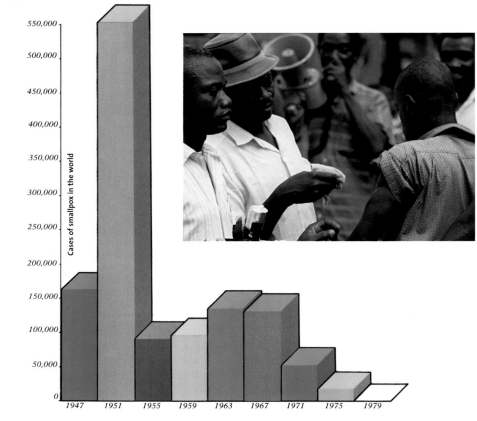

death would occur in the pustular stage of the disease. Once the disease was caught antibiotics were given to try to prevent secondary infection of the pustules by skin bacteria (see Antibiotics). Good nursing was crucial and great care was taken of the mouth, eyes, ears, and skin.

Prevention and eradication

An English doctor, Edward Jenner, discovered in the 18th century, from a milkmaid, that people who had been exposed to cows and had contracted the disease cowpox seemed to be immune to the effects of smallpox. He invented successful immunization, but it took half a century for the true value of his method to be recognized by the medical establishment. Cowpox is caused by a virus called vaccinia, which is very similar to smallpox. By building up antibodies to the milder illness cowpox, the body then has antibodies that work against the smallpox virus (see Vaccinations). However, vaccination was not the prime method by which the disease was eradicated. After all, vaccinated people could still get the disease, and if it was a mild form it might not be recognized and they would be free to roam about and infect other people.

In the mid-1960s, smallpox was to be found in about 50 countries, and no country was entirely free from the disease because of the increased amount of international air travel. By the early 1970s, about 20 countries were still dogged by smallpox; the last major outbreak of the disease was finally eliminated from the Horn of Africa in 1977. The success of the eradication campaign depended upon rapid diagnosis and isolation of cases. This was successful in developed countries, but trained medical personnel were few in the Horn of Africa. Despite these difficulties in this and other parts of the world, the World Health Organization was able to educate the population well enough to recognize the disease and isolate known cases effectively.

See also: **Infection and infectious diseases**

Smart drug

A "smart" drug or "cognitive enhancer" allegedly improves the mental ability of the person who takes it. Smart drugs are also called "nootropics," a term from the Greek words *noos*, meaning "mind," and *tropos*, meaning "change."

Smart drugs were developed in the hope of treating people with neurological disorders such as Alzheimer's disease or patients recovering from a stroke. The symptoms of Alzheimer's disease include confusion, personality change, and gradual memory loss. Examinations of the brains of deceased people who had Alzheimer's disease found that neurons or nerve cells were killed off, including those containing the substance acetylcholine, a neurotransmitter that carries nerve signals around the body. Some scientists believe that acetylcholine might be a neurotransmitter associated with memory. In the United States drugs such as donepezil, galantamine, and rivastigmine may for a time inhibit the body's breakdown of newly formed acetylcholine. They do not, however, cure, stop, or delay the progress of Alzheimer's disease.

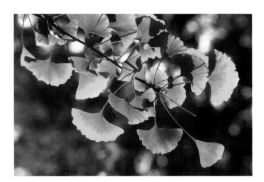

▲ *Ginkgo biloba claims to boost memory, alertness, and learning.*

A stroke is caused by the interruption of the flow of oxygen-carrying blood to the brain. It can result in paralysis or death, but in less severe cases causes memory loss and impairment of thought processes. Doctors reasoned that since blood starvation caused these problems, administering hydergine, derived from the fungus ergot, would encourage blood flow and could help sufferers regain their memory. Some researchers believed that if drugs could be used to help treat people suffering from brain- or memory-related illnesses, they could also be used to enhance the mental capabilities of healthy people. A range of smart drugs quickly developed, which became available through health food shops and mail-order companies, and by prescription. In 2003, there were between 100 and 150 smart drugs available; all claimed to boost cognitive functions. However, conventional medical belief was that the drugs were not effective in this way.

What are smart drugs?

Smart drugs include chemical substances, natural extracts, and nutrients. Among the natural cognitive enhancers are the Chinese herb ma-huang, ginkgo biloba (an extract from the leaves of the ginkgo tree), and BR-16A (an herbal preparation of some 20 ingredients from India). Manufactured pharmaceuticals include piracetam, hydergine, and linopirdine. Smart nutrients included dimethylaminoethanol (DMAE), which occurs in anchovies and sardines; and acetyl-L-carnitine (ALC), an amino acid (an ingredient of proteins) found in milk. Amino acids, such as taurine, are also the "enhancing" ingredients in smart drinks.

Despite the increasing availability of smart drugs and the endorsements they have received from a wide range of scientists and users, critics believe that there is not enough scientific evidence to indicate whether these substances work, or if they are safe. Many of the studies that have been used to prove that cognitive enhancers are effective were based on research carried out on animals such as mice and rats, not people; critics argue that it is difficult to judge how valid these results are with regard to people. Skeptics also argue that the brain of a healthy individual already carries the optimum levels of neurotransmitters, and adding more "fuel" to a healthy brain will not make it perform any better. In the United States, however, some educationalists recommend smart drugs in the treatment of people with Down syndrome and claim that they have seen significant mental development in their students.

See also: Alzheimer's disease; Drug abuse

Smell

Of all the senses, smell is the most evocative; the slightest scent can start a rush of long-forgotten memories. Complex yet primitive, it retains its intimate associations with pleasure and warns of possible danger.

Why is it that if one stays near a smell, the odor fades away until one is almost unaware of it?

This is called adaptation, and is characteristic of our sense of smell, though hearing and touch to some extent show the same phenomenon. If signals persist in coming from the smell receptors in the nose for some time, they are progressively ignored by the part of the brain that sorts them out. This fits in with the function of smell as a warning system.

Do children have a more acute sense of smell than adults?

Yes. The sensitivity of the smell receivers in the nose is at its maximum in childhood and gradually declines through adult life. This is compensated for by the progressively richer associations which smells can evoke as experiences increase.

When a friend quit smoking she remarked that her sense of smell improved. Does smoking really cause such a difference?

A common cause of a diminished sense of smell is heavy smoking, because smoke dries the delicate smelling apparatus and causes a mild inflammation in that part of the nose. The overall effect is to make sensitive-smell receivers much less efficient. When a person quits smoking, the smelling apparatus rapidly returns to normal, and it can be quite a dramatic change.

Do blind people have an enhanced sense of smell?

No. This point has been investigated by researchers who found that blind people's sense of smell is no more acute than sighted people's; neither are any of their other senses enhanced.

The sense of smell is probably the oldest and the least understood of the five senses. During evolution, smell retained connections with parts of the brain that interpret emotional responses and link smells to emotions. The sense of smell also plays an important role in sexual attraction, though this has become considerably muted during human evolutionary development. Its most important roles are those of a warning system and information gatherer, to warn of danger and give valuable information about the outside world.

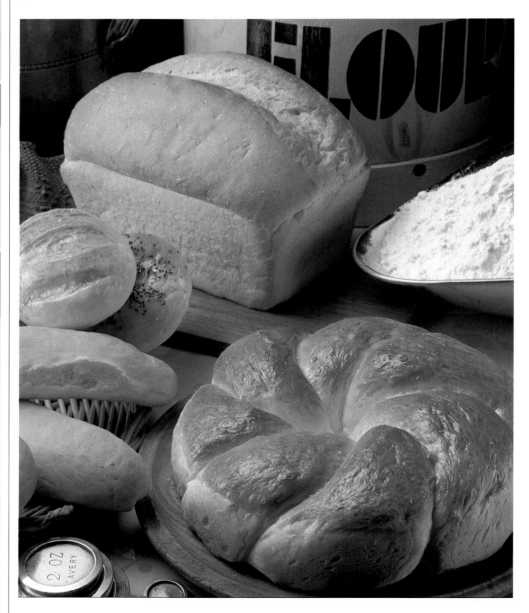

▲ *The fragrance of freshly baked bread makes it irresistible. No food aroma better illustrates how smell enhances taste.*

How do we smell things?

As with many organs in the body, the smelling apparatus is duplicated and each circuit acts independently.

The sensory receptors for smell are found in the roof of the nasal cavity, just beneath the frontal lobes of the brain. This is called the olfactory area and is tightly packed with millions of small cells (the olfactory cells). Each olfactory cell has about a dozen fine hairs, or cilia, which project into a layer of mucus. The mucus keeps the cilia moist and acts as a trap for odorous molecules, and the cilia effectively enlarge the area of each olfactory cell and thereby increase our sensitivity to smells (see Mucus).

It is not clearly understood how minute amounts of chemical substances trigger and stimulate the olfactory cells, but it is known that these substances dissolve in the mucus fluids, stick to the cilia, and then cause the cells to fire electrical signals. Each one of the enormous numbers of olfactory receptor cells carries one or at most a few different kinds of receptor sites. There are approximately 1,000 types of receptor sites, and each one will accept, lock onto, and respond to only one single type of chemically-related odorant molecule. The huge range of odorant molecules are differentiated by the specific chemical groups they carry. In this way, the brain receives information enabling it to discriminate between thousands of different odors.

Olfactory nerve fibers channel these signals across the bone of the skull to the two olfactory bulbs in the brain, where the information is gathered, processed, and then passed through a complicated circuitry of nerve endings to the cerebral cortex. Here the message is identified and the smell becomes a conscious fact.

What is it we smell?

To have an odor, a substance must give off particles of the chemical of which it is made. This type of substance is generally chemically complex. Simple chemical substances, such as salt, do not have a smell, or have only a faint trace of odor.

The particles of a substance must remain in the air in a gaseous form in order to be swept into the nostrils and to the mucus surrounding the cilia. Once in the nostrils, they must be able to dissolve in the mucus for the olfactory apparatus to detect them. Substances that give off gas easily, such as gasoline, are usually very odorous because high concentrations of the chemicals are able to reach the cells.

Wetness also heightens smells. As the water evaporates from the substance, it carries particles of the substance into the air. Perfumes are structured in such a way that they are chemically complex and easily give off gas that can be breathed into the nose and hence into the mucus around the cilia.

▼ *An herb garden is not simply a source of culinary flavorings: its variety of fragrances—from the pungent to the sweet—can provide a relaxing environment.*

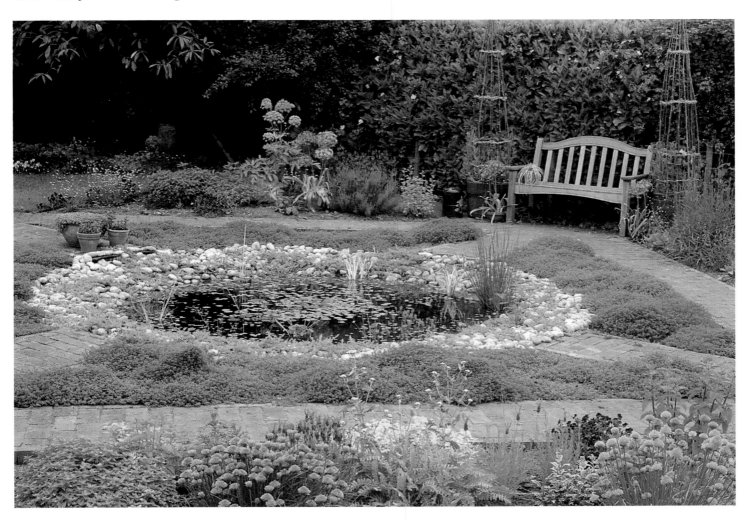

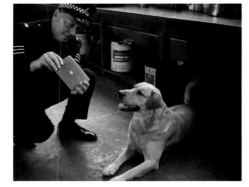

▲ *Animals are extremely sensitive to smells. For example, dogs can be trained to sniff out marijuana.*

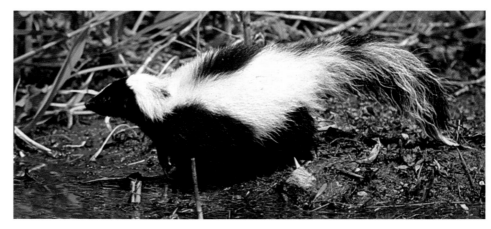

▲ *Skunks defend themselves by emitting a stench sufficient to deter most enemies.*

Purpose of the sense of smell

In humans, the sense of smell appears to have four main purposes: it stimulates the salivary glands in preparation for eating; it has an important role in sexual attraction; it serves as a basic warning system; and it gathers information concerning the world about us.

In the animal world, greater dependence on the sense of smell for survival has given it more specific purposes; locating food, detecting an enemy, and choosing a mate are just a few examples.

The purposes of the human sense of smell have become less defined, because through the ages people have gradually become less dependent on it. Our main senses of vision, hearing, and touch have developed further to provide people with the more accurate information that our higher intelligence requires from the world around them.

The continuing popularity of perfumes for both sexes illustrates that smell has a central but primitive role in the complexities of sexual attraction. This initial attraction between two people is dependent on a number of factors, and the individual smell of a person, known as pheromones, makes a persuasive contribution. Subconsciously, a personal scent helps someone to form an opinion about the other person. If the visual attraction between two people is very strong, but one of the two finds the smell of the other unpleasant, then this is very likely to be a deciding factor in the continuance of the relationship.

A sense of smell also serves as a warning system and gives a person a stream of information about his or her environment. It can be used to determine whether meat is good or bad, whether milk has soured, whether something is burning, or even whether the local wheat crop has been gathered. Although it is extremely sensitive to small quantities of odorous substances, the human sense of smell is not very efficient at detecting differences in the intensity of a smell. Intensity may have to change by a third before the difference is noticeable. In contrast, visual apparatus can detect a 1 percent change in the intensity of light. As a warning and information-gathering system, a sense of smell does not need to notice changes in intensity; it needs to notice only if a scent is actually there. When there is a need to experience as much of a smell as possible, people tend to sniff. This greatly increases the amount of air reaching the smell receivers at the top of the nose, giving them the best chance to sample the new smell.

Links between smell and taste

People are not always aware of the close link between the sense of taste and the sense of smell. However, when someone is suffering from a cold, it is usually noticed that not only has the sense of smell temporarily disappeared, but food has no discernible taste until the cold has cleared up (see Taste).

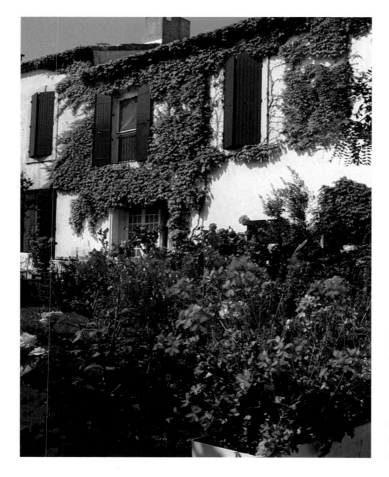

◄ *Natural scents such as the fragrances in a springtime country garden, or the bracing intoxication of the sea air, can be appreciated as much by a sense of smell as by any of the other senses.*

Easy-to-grow fragrant herbs and flowers
Fragrant herbs:
Apothecary's rose (*Rosa gallica officinalis*)
Lemon balm (*Melissa officinalis*)
Lemon verbena (*Aloysia triphylla*)
Rosemary (*Rosmarinus officinalis*)
Lavender (*Lavandula angustifolia*)
Chamomile (*Chamaemelum nobile "Flore Pleno"*)
Fragrant climbers:
Honeysuckle (*Lonicera* spp.)
Jasmine (*Jasminum* ssp.)
Sweet pea (*Lathyrus odoratus*)
Fragrant annuals:
Stock (*Matthiola* spp.)
Lilies (*Lilium* spp.)
Hyacinth (*Hyacinthus* spp.)
Daffodils (*Narcissus* spp.)
Roses (*Rosa* spp.)

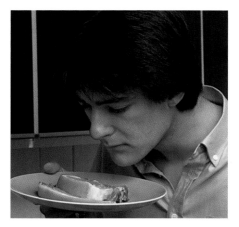

▶ *Smell acts as a warning system: the acrid smell of smoke can alert us to a fire, the smell of burned toast signals to someone to turn off the broiler; the unmistakeable smell of decaying food tells someone that it would be unsafe to eat.*

connection explains why smells are richly endowed with emotional significance. The smell of fresh rain on a summer's day makes people feel happy and invigorated; it may also evoke pleasant memories. The smell of fresh-baked bread will bring on instant pangs of hunger; the scent of perfume may bring anticipation of sexual pleasure. Conversely, unpleasant smells, such as rotten eggs, produce revulsion, and even nausea. Exceptions are the unpleasant smell of a ripe cheese, which actually attracts fervent fans.

Certain smells will bring memories of long-forgotten special occasions flooding back. This is because people tend to remember occasions that have special emotional significance, since the areas of the brain which process memories, and which are essential in their recall, are also closely linked to the limbic system, which, in turn, is linked to the centers in the brain governing the sense of smell.

Smelling disorders
There are two types of smelling disorder: anosmia (the loss of the sense of smell, either complete or partial, either temporary or permanent) and dysosmia (abnormal smell perception).

A decrease in the ability to smell is most commonly due to problems in the nose, as in the common cold, influenza, hay fever, or sinusitis. Heavy smokers also suffer loss of smelling ability, because the delicate smell tissue dries up (see Smoking).

Head injuries, even minor ones, can cause a loss of the sense of smell. This occurs when the delicate olfactory nerves are either bruised or even sheared off by the knock on the head. The loss of smell can be permanent and may affect only one nostril or both (see Head and Head Injuries).

Diseases within the skull can also be associated with a loss of smell, though these are not very common. A tumor or aneurysm pressing on the olfactory nerves may impair the sense of smell, or temporarily interrupt the ability to smell. Meningitis and internal hemorrhaging may also affect the sense of smell.

Dysosmia sometimes occurs as a feature of severe depression or schizophrenia; sufferers can be plagued by illusory unpleasant odors. Similar delusions can also occur in some forms of epilepsy and during drying-out periods after severe alcohol addiction.

Much of what people think of as taste is really smell. In fact, the sense of smell is 10,000 times more sensitive than that of taste. The taste buds in the tongue monitor relatively crude sensations of salt, sweet, sour, and bitter, while the more sophisticated taste sensations are manufactured by smell receivers in the nose. Faint vapors of whatever we are eating drift into the nasal cavity where the smell receptors add more detail to the information given by the taste buds. When the nose is blocked—for example, when someone has a cold—gas and vapors cannot flow over the receiver cells; he or she cannot smell anything and can taste only cruder tastes.

Smell, emotions, and memory
The part of the brain that analyzes messages coming from the receiver cells in the nose is closely connected with the limbic system, a part of the brain that deals with emotions, mood, and memory. It is called the primitive brain, sometimes even the smelling brain. The

Smell and the visually impaired
For people who are blind or partially sighted, smell is an important sense. However, a blind person does not have an improved sense of smell; rather he or she tends to rely on a sense of smell, and get more information from it, than a sighted person. One of the ways that a

blind or partially sighted person can enjoy the sense of smell is to walk or sit in an aromatic garden filled either with herbs or scented flowers. It can become an important and pleasurable part of daily life. The person may not be able to see the flowers but can touch the foliage and smell the various fragrances of the blooms. There are many sweetly fragrant plants that flourish in all seasons and exotic plants that are at their best in hot and tropical climates. Humidity and moist air release more fragrance from the scent glands of a flower, and blind and partially sighted people who live in regions which are both hot and humid will be able to appreciate a well-planned scented garden.

Creating an aromatic garden

When masses of plants are grouped in flower beds the full effect of their fragrance can be enjoyed. Just one or two plants do not create enough of an impact. However, there are some single plants that emit overpowering fragrances. The scented gardenia *Gardenia jasminoides* has been used in the creation of many famous perfumes and is relatively easy to grow in the right climate. A shrub called Daphne (*Daphne* spp.) has a sweet and strong smell. Frangipani are heavy with the scent of orange blossom and honey, particularly a variety called *Hymenosporum flavum*. A night-scented jasmine, *Cestrum nocturnum*, has tubular clusters of waxen green stars that give out an overpowering scent in the evening. Sweet peas are always fragrant, and make an attractive as well as fragrant addition to a garden. The climbers honeysuckle and jasmine and ginger plants have delightful fragrances that most people would find irresistible.

Roses are almost automatically associated with floral fragrance, but because there are many modern varieties that have no fragrance at all, it is important to check at the garden store when buying either a standard or a climbing rose for a scented garden.

There are many trees and shrubs with scented foliage and flowers that will enhance any garden for the visually impaired; for example, the lemonwood, *Pittosporum eugenifolium*, flowers freely, and after it has rained, the air is filled with the cloying scent of honey.

An herb garden bed planted with lavender, lemon thyme, marjoram, wild bergamot, golden sage, lady's mantle, and sage not only will bring pleasure to a blind person but is also practical. Many herbs have household uses and culinary uses as well as having an attractive appearance. People who have visual impairments and do not have a garden can grow scented herbs in containers. The beneficial effects of even a small herb garden can be immense.

SENSE OF SMELL

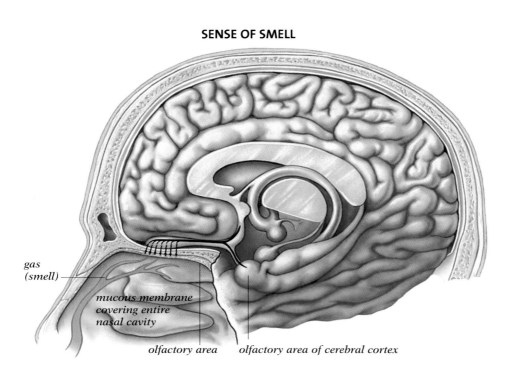

gas (smell)

mucous membrane covering entire nasal cavity

olfactory area

olfactory area of cerebral cortex

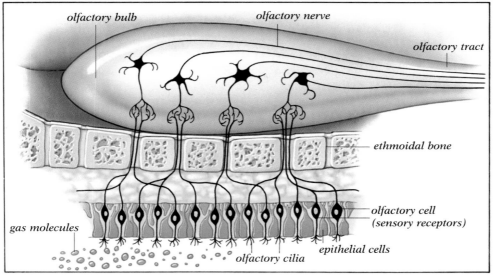

olfactory bulb

olfactory nerve

olfactory tract

ethmoidal bone

olfactory cell (sensory receptors)

gas molecules

epithelial cells

olfactory cilia

▲ *Gaseous substances are dissolved in the mucus surrounding the cilia. A biochemical process then takes place that stimulates the olfactory cells into electrical activity. These messages are passed across the ethmoidal bone via sensory nerve fibers, and into the olfactory bulb. Here the information is processed and then it is passed along the complex circuitry of the olfactory nerves to the cerebral cortex. At this point people become aware of the smell.*

See also: Common cold; Epilepsy; Nose; Sinusitis

Smoking

The phrase "dying for a cigarette" is brutally apt. Fatal smoking-related diseases constitute a genuine epidemic and, unusually, it is one that is solely in the hands of the potential victims to eradicate.

Questions and Answers

Will nicotine chewing gum or patches help me quit smoking?

Yes. Trials have shown that nicotine chewing gum and transdermal patches do reduce the craving for a cigarette, which is a common cause of failure in the first weeks of trying to give up smoking. They are effective antismoking aids worth trying.

I have tried, but I cannot give up smoking. Can I do anything to reduce the risk of getting a smoking-related disease?

Yes, there are several things that are worth doing. First, move down the scale of tar content step by step from high, to middle to high, to middle, and so on until you are smoking low-tar cigarettes. Second, on no account smoke any more cigarettes than your daily minimum. Use filter-tipped cigarettes; the benefit is not dramatic but it's enough to make some difference. Third, try not to inhale. Even though some of the nicotine is absorbed through the mouth and throat there are still advantages. Try to smoke less by gradually increasing the interval between cigarettes, leaving very long stubs, taking the cigarette out of your mouth between puffs, and increasing the interval between puffs.

My five-year-old daughter has asthma. I smoked very heavily during pregnancy. Did this cause her condition?

Children of mothers who smoke during pregnancy do have health disadvantages. They have a lower level of resistance that makes them more prone to infectious diseases, and they are usually slower to develop both physically and mentally. However, there is no evidence that asthma in children is caused by the mother smoking when pregnant.

Smoking the dried leaves of the tobacco plant in the form of cigarettes or cigars or in pipes was introduced into England around the middle of the 16th century by explorers and adventurers who had found the practice established in the New World. Consumption of tobacco in industrialized countries continued to increase until 1973, and then began to fall, but it remains among the most common habits in the Western world. It is an extremely dangerous habit with no less than lethal consequences for a very large proportion of those who indulge in it. And it is an addiction that is difficult to break.

Why do people smoke?

People smoke for a wide variety of reasons. Once they have smoked their first few experimental cigarettes, which can cause coughing, nausea, and sometimes vomiting, most smokers get pleasure from the taste and aroma of tobacco and tobacco smoke. They may also get pleasure from the whole ritual of lighting up: from handling cigarettes, a lighter, or matches; from the action of inhaling; and from watching the smoke curl upward.

Smokers make two claims for their habit: first, that smoking sedates them, or settles their nerves, when they need sedating; second, that it acts as a stimulant when they need to work. Evidence has shown that these effects are due to nicotine and that both these claims are true, depending on the dose, on what the smoker is doing, and on his or her particular psychological and physical makeup (see Sedatives; Stimulants). There is also a true physical addiction to nicotine so that when deprived of the drug the person concerned suffers from unpleasant

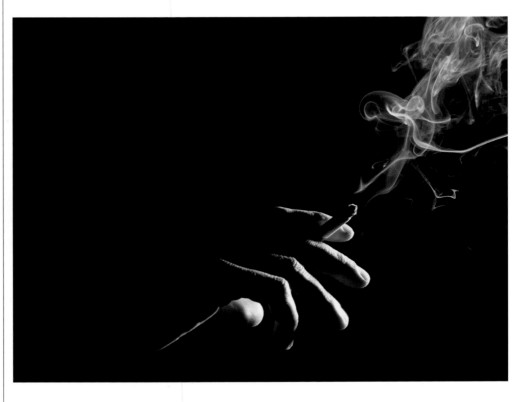

▲ *The sight and smell of cigarettes is unpleasant, but far more important than these aesthetic considerations, cigarettes are dangerous to health.*

Questions and Answers

How efficient are filters in actually removing harmful substances from cigarette smoke?

Putting a filter on a cigarette certainly reduces the tar and nicotine your body absorbs. In addition, there is evidence that people who smoke filter-tipped cigarettes are at less risk of getting lung cancer. So there certainly is some advantage. However, the benefit is certainly not so great that it is safe to smoke filter cigarettes. Probably the best that can be said for them is that if you cannot give up altogether, they are a little less dangerous than nonfilter brands.

Why do doctors tell you that if you must smoke, smoke only the first half of the cigarette?

For two reasons. The first is that the tar concentration in the bottom half of the cigarette, and particularly in the stub, is very much greater than in the top half. If you smoke only the top half of the cigarette, or at least leave a long stub, you are doing yourself a favor. The second reason is that any change in your habit which has the effect of decreasing the total amount that you actually smoke will benefit you by a similar amount. That is why those who have not been able to give up are strongly encouraged to at least try to make do with only half a cigarette at a time.

I stopped smoking five years ago. Will my lungs have returned to a normally healthy state?

That really depends on how long and how heavily you smoked before you gave up the habit. What is certain is that further damage to your lungs—and other parts of your body—stops from the time you give it up. It is clear that there is an improvement in lung capacity and your chances of getting either lung cancer or bronchitis drop. After 12 to 15 years of not smoking, the risk of developing lung cancer is the same as if you had never smoked.

physical withdrawal symptoms which are relieved only by a further dose (see Nicotine). Dependence on smoking may be psychological as well as physical; smokers miss whatever enjoyment they get from smoking but do not really need it. Often, too, smoking has become such an ingrained habit that the smoker has a cigarette almost without being aware of it.

Some people smoke because they associate smoking with sociability. To offer and to take cigarettes establishes a bond between people. To the shy and introverted, it offers something for them to do with their hands and makes them appear self-confident. The smoker may smoke as much to be one of the company as to get pleasure from smoking. The pleasure comes from being with others and not from the cigarette.

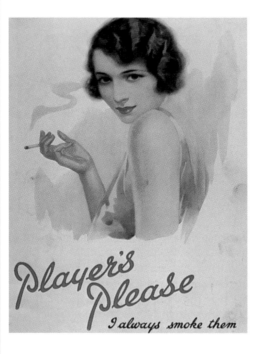

The climate of opinion prevailing is an important factor in determining smoking, and over the last few years much has been done to try to discourage smokers. In more and more countries, smoking is now banned in public places such as movie theaters and subways. Many restaurants, bars, and places of work have adopted a no-smoking policy and it is no longer assumed that everyone wishes to be in

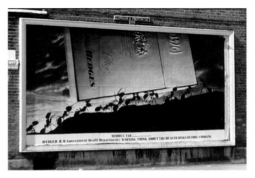

▼▲ *In the past, cigarette advertisers freely promoted the image of smoking as a sophisticated, and even, by associating it with the rigors of outdoor life, healthy activity. Now that there is evidence of the risks smokers run, and strict curbs have been placed on cigarette advertising, things are not so simple for the tobacco companies. They now have to advertise their products more obliquely, and with health warnings attached that sometimes loom larger than the advertisement itself. The sponsorship of sport is one of the principal means the industry uses to promote its product, although there are now moves to ban the practice.*

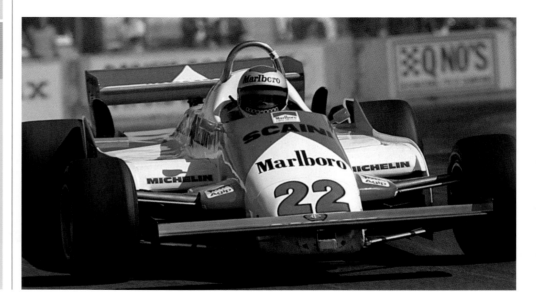

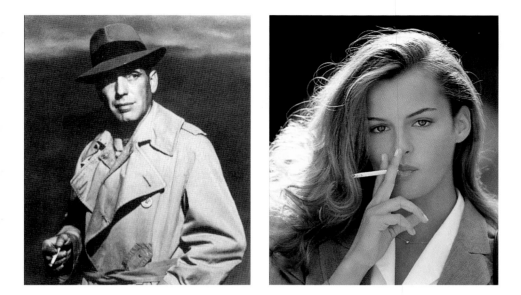

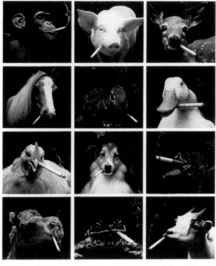

It Looks Just As Stupid When You Do It.

▲ *The glamorous image that smoking developed in film and fashion concealed the cost in health. Humphrey Bogart died from throat cancer.*

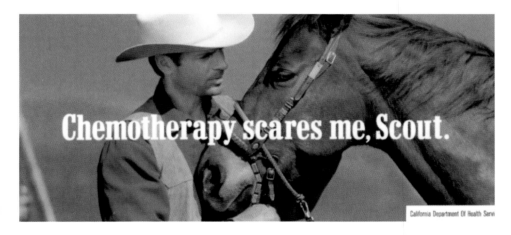

▲ *Showing animals smoking and looking rather silly was meant to appeal to young people to make them realize how uncool smoking can appear to other people.*

◄ *This controversial billboard advertisement attempts to inspire fear in would-be smokers by using well-known images and twisting the text to get the message across.*

▼ *Antitobacco advertising is aimed at teens, who are most vulnerable to starting smoking. This stained-glass image was part of an antismoking campaign in 2003.*

smoke-filled environments. Some states are now pressing, and winning, claims for damages against the tobacco industry (which is worth billions of dollars) in order to finance the growing costs of health care resulting from smoking-related diseases.

Factors in starting smoking

There are strong connections between children's smoking and the smoking habits of their parents and older brothers and sisters. This is not surprising when the strength of family bonds and the desire of small children to be like their elders is taken into account. Children in the early years at school usually disapprove of the tobacco habit intensely. By the early teens, however, they are ready to experiment with smoking, and this is because of the strong identification formed at an earlier stage between drinking and smoking and being and acting like an adult.

What's wrong with smoking?

In Britain, shortly after the end of World War II, Professor A. Bradford Hill and Dr. Richard Doll published the first of a series of papers leading to the inescapable conclusion that cigarette smoking was the major factor in the rising incidence of lung cancer (see Cancer; Lung and Lung Diseases). They began with a retrospective study, in which they investigated a large number of patients with cancer of the lung and compared them with a carefully matched control group who did not have this form of cancer. After they compared a number of factors that might have a bearing on the cause of this disease, the only great difference to emerge

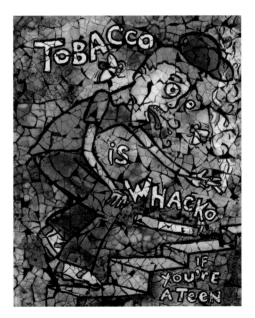

AGE-ADJUSTED DEATH RATES FOR SELECTED CANCER SITES, 2000

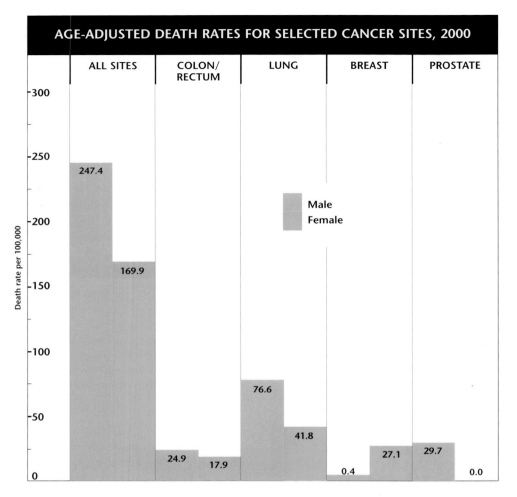

	ALL SITES	COLON/RECTUM	LUNG	BREAST	PROSTATE
	■ Male ■ Female				
Male	247.4	24.9	76.6	0.4	29.7
Female	169.9	17.9	41.8	27.1	0.0

Death rate per 100,000 — 300, 250, 200, 150, 100, 50, 0

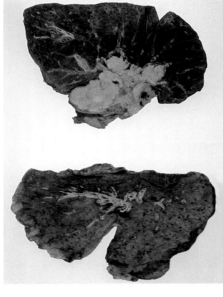

▲ *The large, visible mass of white tissue (top) is a cancer in the lung of a smoker. The lung beneath it is healthy and free from this deadly disease.*

◄ *The table shows a snapshot of the year 2000. The table shows death rates for the four most prevalent types of cancer, divided into male and female sufferers, and adjusted for age.*

was that the smoking habits of the two groups varied. Only one in 200 male lung cancer patients were nonsmokers, indicating smoking as the cause. The same type of statistics appeared among studies of women. Furthermore, there appeared to be a relationship between the risk of getting lung cancer and the number of cigarettes a person smoked.

The problem with this kind of retrospective investigation is that people's memory, especially if they are sick, is inclined to be faulty. Bradford Hill and Doll therefore set up an investigation that would study the prospective health of smokers. They had 25,000 British doctors give details of their smoking habits as well as a variety of other relevant information. All the doctors were apparently well and had no reason to lie, and gave details of present smoking habits rather than the sometimes faulty recollections of past smoking. As the years passed, some of these doctors died; Doll and Bradford Hill investigated the cause of death in each case. Some of the deaths were from lung cancer and two facts emerged quite clearly. First, there was a very clear relationship between cigarette smoking and lung

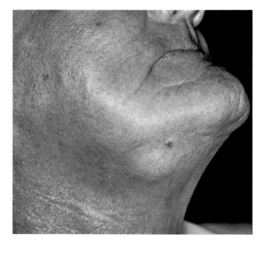

▲ *Simple and quick treatment is not possible to remove a smoking-related cancer of the jaw.*

cancer. Second, the chances of dying from the disease increased with increasing cigarette consumption.

Since then a mass of evidence confirming these results has poured in from all over the world. It also soon became clear that cigarette smoking was an important factor in causing other diseases, of which the most important are chronic bronchitis (see Bronchitis) and coronary heart disease (see Heart Disease). The end result was the demonstration of two important facts: first, cigarette smokers live, on average, shorter lives than nonsmokers; and second, giving up smoking removes this excess risk in proportion to the amount of time that has elapsed since giving up.

In addition to the main diseases already mentioned above, there is evidence that cigarette smoking can cause other types of pulmonary disorders (see Pulmonary Disorders); delays the healing of gastric ulcers (see Ulcers); is a major cause of various cancers of the mouth, voice box, esophagus, and bladder; and leads to a degree of skin wrinkling appropriate to nonsmokers who are 20 years older (see Wrinkles). It may not be widely appreciated that it is not nicotine that causes the harm

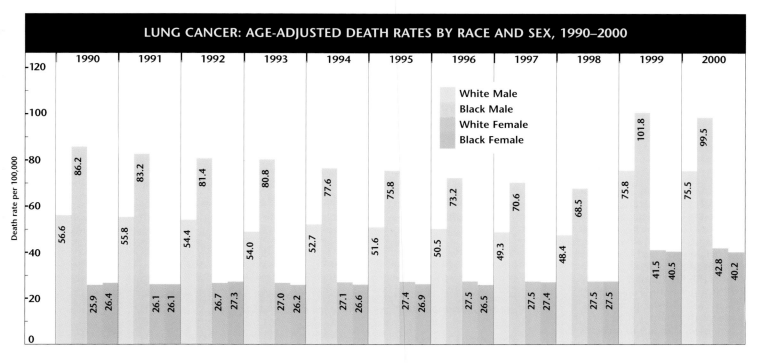

LUNG CANCER: AGE-ADJUSTED DEATH RATES BY RACE AND SEX, 1990–2000

Death rate per 100,000

Legend:
White Male
Black Male
White Female
Black Female

Year	White Male	Black Male	White Female	Black Female
1990	56.6	86.2	25.9	26.4
1991	55.8	83.2	26.1	26.1
1992	54.4	81.4	26.7	27.3
1993	54.0	80.8	27.0	26.2
1994	52.7	77.6	27.1	26.6
1995	51.6	75.8	27.4	26.9
1996	50.5	73.2	27.5	26.5
1997	49.3	70.6	27.5	27.4
1998	48.4	68.5	27.5	27.5
1999	75.8	101.8	41.5	40.5
2000	75.5	99.5	42.8	40.2

from smoking. Smoking is dangerous because of the toxic substances in the vaporized tar. Cigarette tars contain some 3,000 different chemical substances of which several are carcinogenic and several cause other forms of damage to the body.

There are other factors about smoking that are worth knowing. Among nonsmokers, only about one in five will not reach retirement age; but for smokers of over 25 cigarettes a day, two in five will not reach retirement age. The death rate for smokers is much higher among those who inhale than among those who do not; the earlier you start smoking the greater the risk; and the more you smoke the greater the risk. According to findings in the United States, the use of filter-tipped cigarettes does slightly reduce the risk of lung cancer. For pipe (only) and cigar (only) smokers the risk of getting lung cancer is small, provided they do not inhale, although the chance is greater than for nonsmokers.

Effects on nonsmokers

There is an increasing amount of evidence that smoke inhaled by nonsmokers is harmful to their health. It has been shown that the smoke drifting up from the burning end of the cigarette contains twice as much tar as that inhaled by the smoker.

Concern about the effects of second-hand smoke and the rights of nonsmokers has led to changes in attitudes and even in the law in some cases. Nonsmoking areas are now common in public places and in the workplace; and many theaters, restaurants, and public transport facilities ban smoking altogether. There is also an increasing awareness about the risks to an

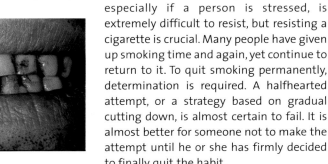

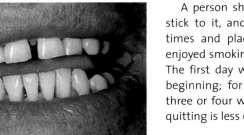

▲ *Nicotine badly stains the teeth, but if you stop smoking, your teeth can once again be sparkling clean.*

unborn baby if a woman smokes during pregnancy (see Pregnancy). Smoking mothers have higher rates of miscarriages, stillbirths (see Stillbirth), and infant deaths than nonsmoking mothers.

How to stop smoking

Giving up is not easy. There are no miracle cures, no magic methods, no shortcuts, and no foolproof formulas. Nevertheless it is a battle that can be won and several million people quit smoking every year. For a person to give up something that he or she enjoys and has come to rely on is painful. The temptation to have just one cigarette, especially if a person is stressed, is extremely difficult to resist, but resisting a cigarette is crucial. Many people have given up smoking time and again, yet continue to return to it. To quit smoking permanently, determination is required. A halfhearted attempt, or a strategy based on gradual cutting down, is almost certain to fail. It is almost better for someone not to make the attempt until he or she has firmly decided to finally quit the habit.

A person should plan a campaign, and stick to it, and beware of and avoid the times and places when he or she most enjoyed smoking and break those routines. The first day without smoking is just the beginning; for many people it can take three or four weeks, or even longer, before quitting is less of a struggle.

See also: **Arteries and artery disease; Heart attack; Miscarriage**

Snakebite

Thousands of venomous snakebites occur each year, but people can take steps to avoid being bitten. If treatment for snakebite is given quickly, in the form of intravenous fluids and possibly antivenins, recovery is swift.

Although snakes are feared in some countries, in Southeast Asia they are believed to be powerful spirits that bring good luck. A common misconception is that all snakes are dangerous. In fact, species that are venomous form a very small part of the snake population.

In the United States, deaths from snakebite are extremely rare. There are roughly 7,000 snakebites each year, leading to only 15 deaths. Almost 3,000 of this total of snakebites occur in people who handle snakes. The chance of surviving a venomous snakebite is thus about 99.8 percent. Deaths are far more common, however, in less developed countries. It has been estimated that between 30,000 and 40,000 people die worldwide from snakebites each year, 75 percent of them in India. Myanmar (formerly Burma) has the highest mortality rate: 15.4 deaths per 100,000 population per annum (see Bites and Stings).

Venomous snakes

Venomous snakes are characterized by the structure of their fangs. For example, the African boomslang has fangs at the back of the mouth, each bearing a groove down which venom flows. The cobra has grooved fangs at the front of the mouth. Rattlesnakes and vipers have the most sophisticated biting apparatus; the fangs are hinged, and, when not in use, fold back along the roof of the mouth. The toxicity of snake venom varies. The world's most venomous snakes are the sea snakes (*Hydrophidae*), which have a venom 100 times as powerful as that of a king cobra; the poison of the cobra can kill an adult in minutes if it strikes at the face.

The amount of venom injected by a snake during an attack is significant. Cobra venom is

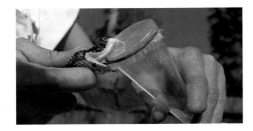

▲ *The process of extracting venom is called milking.*

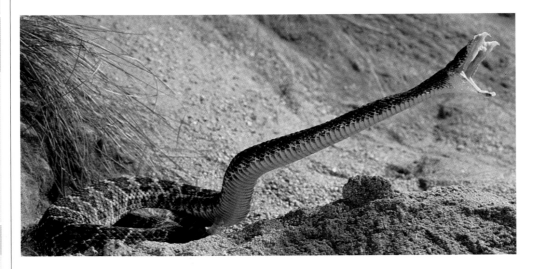

▲ *The western diamondback rattlesnake, found in the United States from Texas to California, is extremely dangerous—not only because of the toxicity of its venom, but also because of its aggressiveness and speed. Because of improved methods of treatment, fatalities are rare.*

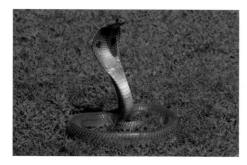

▲ *The cobra is revered in some parts of the East, but its bite is feared everywhere in the world.*

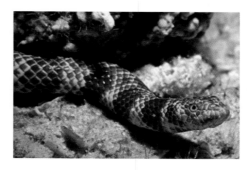

▲ *Sea snakes are among the most venomous snakes. They live in tropical parts of the Indian and Pacific oceans.*

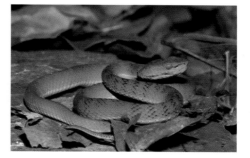

▲ *The deadly Pope's pit viper is found only in Asia: its venom acts on both the blood and the muscles.*

five times more powerful than viper venom, but vipers have a more efficient injection technique than cobras. The habits of the snake and the vulnerability of its victim are relevant factors; for example, the cobra is very alert and is found in areas where many people go barefoot, making the snake doubly dangerous. Vipers, on the other hand, are sluggish and easily trodden on, so the majority of attacks are the result of inattention on the part of the walker.

Symptoms

The action of snake venom depends on the species. Generally speaking, the venom may affect the body in one of three ways. It may cause hemorrhage, clotting, or inhibition of clotting, or tissue damage; it may affect the central nervous system or the heart; or it may release histamine and bradykinin from the tissues, causing pain or swelling. The main effect of viper venom is often to stop the blood from clotting. Pain and swelling result and in some cases tissue is lost at the site of the bite.

Cobra venom, on the other hand, is neurotoxic; it attacks the nervous system, causing paralysis (see Paralysis), especially of the respiratory system, and failure of the swallowing mechanism.

Sea snakes inject an extremely powerful venom that breaks down muscle tissues in the body and causes the body's vital organs, such as the kidneys, to fail (see Kidneys and Kidney Diseases). An attack by a snake, however, is usually a defensive measure and in about 50 percent of cases little or no venom is injected.

Treatment

The development of antisnakebite serum (antivenin), which can be injected intravenously or intramuscularly, makes treating snakebite much easier than it used to be, provided that the serum is administered in reasonable time. Sera are made by injecting animals with small amounts of venom to build up antibodies to the poison. The serum derived from the animals' blood will contain these antibodies and can be used to combat the effects of the bite in humans. However, since antivenins are serum from a foreign species, they may cause a reaction in the host, and other drugs need to be given to cover the injection, such as epinephrine or steroids. For this reason, doctors use antivenin serum only with discretion. There is usually a time lag between a snakebite and giving antivenin. However, for most poisonous snakebites, first-aid measures can be taken. Most important, the patient should be reassured, because fear can be a major symptom. The bitten limb should be immobilized and a firm bandage applied, and the patient taken to the hospital, with the body of the snake for identification, if possible. The bite should never be cut into, and the wound should not be sucked to extract the venom; either practice may do more harm than good.

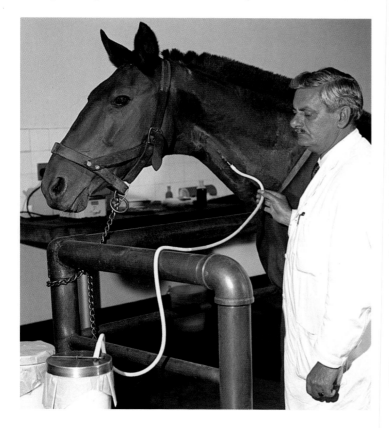

▲ *Animals, particularly horses, are injected with venom, and their blood is then used to make antivenin serum.*

◄ *When a snake strikes, its fangs leave characteristic puncture marks in the skin.*

See also: Hemorrhage; Steroids

Sneezing

I used to sneeze a lot and have a permanently blocked nose, but I found that using a spray I bought from the drugstore helped. I now have to use more and more to get relief. Is it safe to continue?

See your doctor. Many people unwittingly cause permanent damage to the lining of the nose with these preparations, which tend gradually to lose their effectiveness. Your doctor will be able to give you a prescription for a medication which does not damage the nose, or send you to an ear, nose, and throat specialist.

I was told that my heart misses a beat when I sneeze. Is this true?

Not entirely. When you breathe in your heart speeds up and when you breathe out it slows down. The more pronounced the inspiration and expiration, the more your heart speeds up or slows down. Sneezing involves deep inspiration and expiration, so your heart rate may be affected by it. This will not affect your health; it is a normal phenomenon called sinus arrhythmia.

I heard that a girl who couldn't stop sneezing was sent to Switzerland. Why?

Mountain air is free from allergens, so patients with allergic rhinitis may improve in this environment. Sea air may have a similar effect.

I take antihistamines for hay fever. They relieve my symptoms but I hear it is dangerous to drive when taking them. Is this so?

No, unless they make you sleepy. If so, you should reduce the dose or ask your doctor to prescribe a nonsedative preparation. Alcohol also enhances the sedative effects of antihistamines.

Like so many of our reflexes, sneezing is an important mechanism designed to protect the body. It may, however, sometimes be a sign of an abnormal state needing investigation and suitable treatment.

The prime function of the nose is to clean up inspired air—the air we breathe in. The structure of the nose is designed for this function. A coarse sieve of hairs within the nostrils, called the nasal vibrissae, and a finer sieve, the nasal mucosa, line the nostrils with mucus. Both sieves filter out dust and other particles from the incoming air. The sense of smell monitors inspired air, and a reflex action, the sneeze, totally clears the nasal and mouth passages.

The sneezing mechanism

Sneezing is triggered by irritation of the nasal mucosa and results in a sudden, violent expulsion of expiratory gases through the nose and mouth. This outburst carries with it the irritant in the form of droplets, which may be projected up to 30 feet (9 m). During the explosive phase the eyes of the person sneezing close by reflex action.

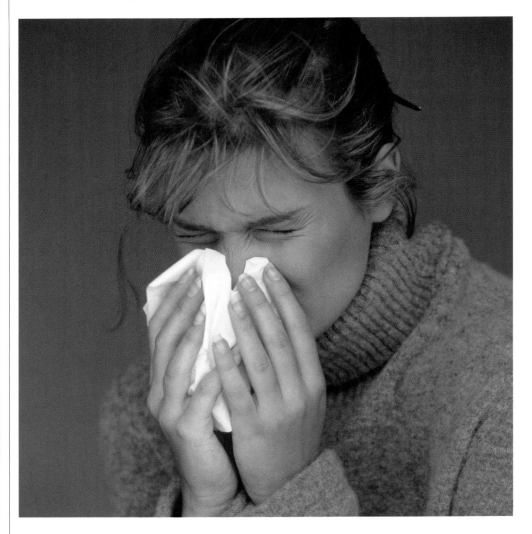

▲ *Always use a handkerchief when you sneeze. A virus can travel from person to person in the droplets, which are often carried a long way by the violence of a sneeze.*

Causes

Sneezing can be a normal reaction to irritants of the nasal mucosa, such as smoke, aerosol sprays, or sudden changes in temperature or humidity. It may even follow a knock on the nose. The common cold is probably the most frequent cause of sneezing (see Common Cold), because the virus and secondary bacterial infection make the nasal mucosa hypersensitive to minor stimuli.

There are, however, conditions in which the nose is irritated abnormally, or in which sneezing is induced by factors that do not affect the majority of people. These include the presence of foreign bodies, and an abnormally sensitive nasal lining.

Foreign bodies

Children are frequently admitted to the hospital when objects, such as beads or peanuts, have become lodged in the nasal passages. Within a few hours the child begins to sneeze as the foreign body irritates the nasal mucosa, secretions are trapped, and infection builds up. This results in a nasal discharge containing pus (see Pus); it also results in bad breath and sometimes intermittent nosebleeds.

Removal of foreign bodies usually requires general anesthesia. The doctor will also check that no other foreign bodies are hidden in the ears, for instance.

Allergic rhinitis

Sneezing is also part of an abnormal reaction to an inhaled substance or allergen, so called because it is allergy-producing. The most common allergens are the grass and tree pollens that are responsible for hay fever, and the droppings of the house dust mite, which are found in most houses and may cause many allergic problems (see Hay Fever).

In a sensitive person antibodies are already attached to certain cells in the nasal mucosa. They are called mast cells. When an allergen enters, the antibodies fuse with them and in so doing tear the membranes of the mast cells. These then disintegrate and release histamine, which is highly irritant and produces an inflammatory response, in which patients are overcome by bouts of violent sneezing and have a profuse watery discharge and nasal obstruction. Treatment involves identification of the particular allergen so that it can be avoided or at least reduced. This is done by skin testing (see Allergies).

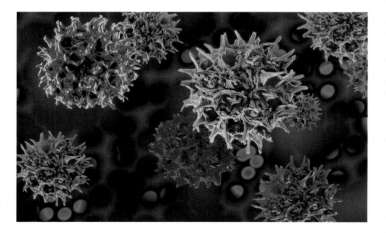

▲ *A greatly magnified computer-generated graphic image of pollen depicts the grains that cause pollen allergy or hay fever.*

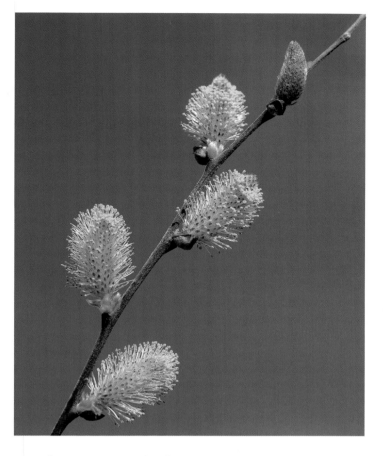

▲ *A close-up picture of willow catkins clearly shows pollen on the long clusters of flowers. Pollen is an allergen that affects people susceptible to hay fever and makes them sneeze.*

Treatment

Three types of drug are in use that control a patient's nasal symptoms. Antihistamines act by blocking the effect of histamine on surrounding cells. Disodium cromoglycate, taken as a spray or in drops, prevents the release of histamine from the mast cells, but is effective only if taken in advance of an attack.

Topical steroids work by suppressing the inflammatory reaction triggered by histamine release. Their activity is confined solely to the nose, and so they are deemed to be safe. When no medicine is effective, the patient may be given desensitizing injections.

Vasomotor rhinitis

A condition that produces symptoms similar to allergic rhinitis, but in which there is no obvious allergen, is called vasomotor rhinitis. There are two types, one of which involves a great deal of sneezing and a watery nasal discharge. Most cases respond to antihistamines and topical steroids, and some may be controlled by oral decongestant preparations, which shrink and soothe the nasal lining. Sneezing and nasal secretions are then reduced and airflow improves.

A few patients may need minor surgery to reduce the amount of nasal lining while at the same time preserving a sense of smell. The procedure is not painful, and improvement can be obvious in a few weeks.

> *See also:* **Breathing; Nose; Steroids; Surgery**

Snoring

Sleeping with the mouth open—whether it's because someone has a cold or has simply fallen asleep in an uncomfortable position—may cause snoring. It's a harmless phenomenon, but can be very irritating to others.

Snoring, breathing heavily through the mouth with a vibrating or snorting noise when asleep, is chronic in as many as one in eight sleepers. The noise can disturb partners and the snorers themselves and in some cases can cause great distress. Snoring can be a symptom of a much more serious condition called sleep apnea, in which breathing repeatedly stops during sleep. This condition can be confirmed by various tests and sleep studies.

The causes of snoring

Snoring is an involuntary act. The characteristic noise is created when, for some reason, the sleeper begins to breathe through his or her mouth, and the muscles of the soft palate and the uvula are allowed to relax. The passage through which air passes is narrowed, and, as the sleeper inhales, the air drawn into the lungs causes the soft palate and the uvula to vibrate. The quality and the intensity of the snoring will be governed by the shape of the mouth, the elasticity of the tissues, and the vigor with which the snorer inhales. Occasionally people snore so vigorously that they wake themselves up, but generally a snorer is oblivious of the noise he or she is making. Because snoring occurs when a person sleeps with the mouth open, a blocked nose or anything obstructing the nasal airways which forces breath out through the mouth will make snoring far more likely. A stuffy nose because of a cold, or enlarged tonsils or adenoids, may make someone

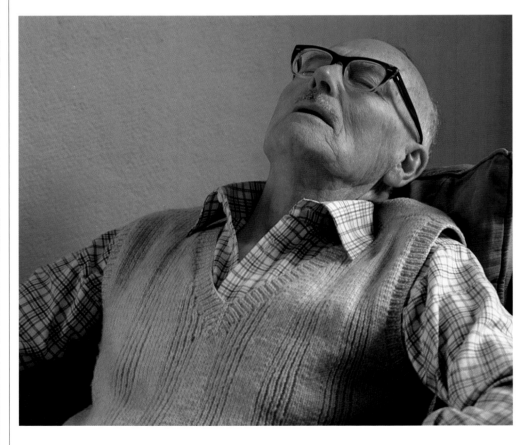

▲ *Falling asleep in a chair is likely to cause someone to snore. The head is thrown back and the mouth opens. This makes breathing through the mouth all too easy.*

likely to breathe through the mouth (see Adenoids; Tonsils). If the muscles of the lower jaw and palate relax in sleep, snoring may start. A person who is sitting up and falls asleep loses control over these muscles and they relax. This is why so many people snore when they fall asleep sitting up on trains or in armchairs. Similarly, a person who lies on his or her back when asleep may also be prone to snoring because the lower jaw drops and the muscles of the palate relax (see Palate).

There have been suggestions that people who are overweight are more likely to snore than their normal counterparts, though it is hard to see why this should be the case. After all, no fat is laid down in the nasal passages to cause obstruction. It has been shown, however, that if a snorer who is overweight loses a few pounds, there is likely to be a reduction of noise caused by snoring, if not a complete cessation of snoring.

The atmosphere where someone is asleep may also have an effect. A very dry, centrally heated room can lead to snoring in a susceptible individual, as can an exceptionally humid environment.

Stopping snoring

Since snoring involves breathing through the mouth in sleep, most forms of treatment to alleviate the condition aim at trying to reestablish breathing through the nose. If someone who does not normally snore develops a cold and is told that he or she has started snoring, all that is needed to be done is to relieve the symptoms of the cold so that he or she can breathe through the nose again. In the same way, treating obstructions such as enlarged adenoids in the nasal airways will relieve, if not cure, the snoring.

Colds and nasal obstructions, however, contribute only to a temporary snoring problem, and other forms of treatment have to be tried in more indeterminate cases. Some measures are commonsense: for example, if people snore when they are sleeping

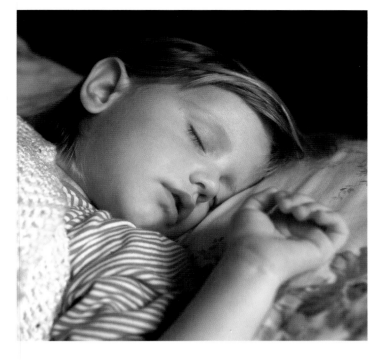

▲ *If children have adenoid problems, they are quite likely to start snoring because the blocked nose, caused by the adenoids, forces them to breathe through the mouth.*

on their back, they need to be persuaded to sleep on their side, or their stomach. There are also exercises designed to keep the mouth closed while the snorer is asleep, for example clenching the teeth for 10 minutes or so before retiring, and these have proved successful in some cases of snoring.

A more modern suggestion for helping persistent snorers involves using a cervical collar—the same type that is used for treating a sprained neck—when going to bed. The rationale is justifiable: snoring is often at its worst when the sufferer is lying on his or her back with the head sagging on the chest. The cervical collar will keep the chin and the lower jaw elevated, and so, it is hoped, prevent snoring from beginning.

Living with a snorer

The irritation that can be engendered by a persistent snorer, who is blissfully ignorant of the noise he or she is making, can be almost unbearable and very distressing. However, there is usually a physical reason for the condition, and it should be possible to relieve it. If snoring continues, earplugs for the other person may be the only solution.

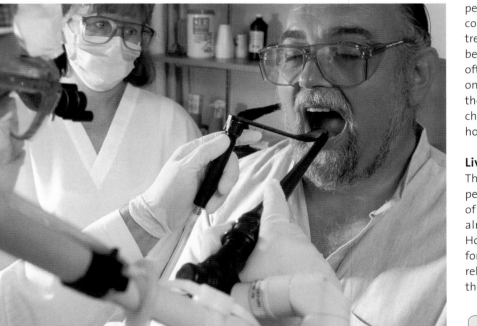

▲ *A doctor performs an assisted urula palatoplasty in his office. This surgical procedure is said to help reduce snoring.*

See also: Breathing; Insomnia; Muscles; Obesity; Sleep and sleep problems; Stress; Weight

Solvent abuse

Called the "silent epidemic," solvent abuse has become one of the most common and preventable forms of substance abuse and kills both children and adolescents. What is solvent abuse, and how can it be prevented?

Solvents are just one of the many harmful poisons that growing numbers of children and adolescents are intentionally abusing to get a feeling of euphoria. Inhalant abuse is akin to playing Russian roulette, and for many people their first experience will also be their last. Out of every 10 deaths caused by inhalant abuse, three of the victims will be first-time users.

Where are solvents found?

Solvents are easily available to everyone from various sources. Ammonia, bleach, and disinfectants can be found in most kitchens; antifreeze, turpentine, and kerosene can be found in the garage; aerosol sprays, felt-tip markers, glues, paints, and rust removers can be found in workshops. School supplies that contain dangerous chemicals include cements and glues, correction fluid, and permanent markers; wood shops may have varnishes and paint remover; graphic arts classes might stock printing inks and computer

▶ *Some manufacturers have changed the chemical composition of their products to reduce the likelihood of solvent abuse. In addition, retailers can display prominent signs warning of the dangers of the practice and back them up by refusing to sell glue to children under the age of 16.*

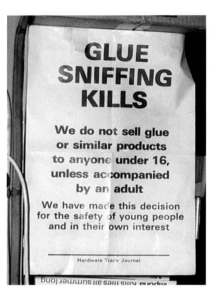

GLUE SNIFFING KILLS

We do not sell glue or similar products to anyone under 16, unless accompanied by an adult

We have made this decision for the safety of young people and in their own interest

Hardware Trade Journal

Is it possible to die from sniffing a bottle of correction fluid?

Yes. Correction fluid is made from the same poisonous chemicals as paint strippers, bleach, and pesticides. Toxic vapors replace the oxygen in the body, and can permanently damage the brain, destroy the kidneys and liver, collapse the lungs, and stop the heart. Anxiety, a sudden scare, or stress, such as might be caused by a frantic parent, can also provoke a cardiac arrest. People can die the first time they try inhalants.

Is it likely that my six-year-old sister sniffs chemicals?

Inhalant abuse is very common. In 2003, the American Academy of Family Physicians revealed that a survey showed that 20 percent of children in middle school and high school have experimented with inhaled substances. They are dangerous because they are cheap and easy to obtain.

How can I tell if my teenage son is using inhalants?

Telltale signs are drunken behavior, a glazed look, and loss of appetite. You may smell a characteristic chemical odor on his breath or clothing, or notice red rashes, spots, or sores around his mouth from chemical contact. Other clues include paint or other stains on the body and clothing, or hidden stashes of solvents.

Is describing solvent abuse tantamount to encouraging it?

No. Prevention campaigns are essential, especially for preadolescents and adolescents. They and their parents must be made aware of the danger of death, burns, and brain damage. Promoting education about inhalant abuse is vital.

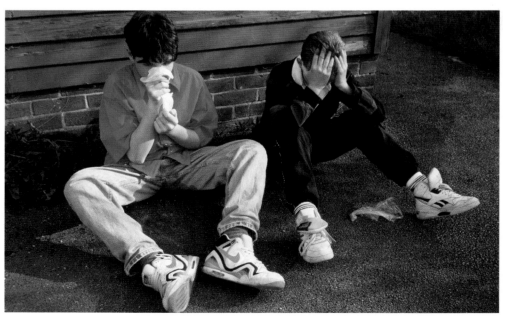

▲ *Young people aged eight to 17 are the main abusers of solvents; those involved often inhale glue vapor by pouring the adhesive into a plastic bag and breathing in and out.*

cleaners; culinary arts students have access to whipping cream cartridges and cans; beauticians are exposed to hair sprays and nail polish remover.

Inhalant victims come from either sex, all ethnic backgrounds, and all economic classes. However, chronic use is most common among young white males. Young people aged eight to 17 are the main abusers; the peak age is 13. Some sniff the solvents, some huff the inhalants directly into their mouths. For preteenage children, solvent abuse is more popular than marijuana.

What are the effects?

When inhaled, most solvents produce effects similar to anesthetics. The user can experience slight stimulation, less inhibition, intoxication, or loss of consciousness. Spray paint and butane damage the peripheral nerves, and cause numbness or tingling sensations. Some people become nauseated, forgetful, and unable to see things clearly. Others may lose control of their body, and the use of arms and legs. Because most inhalants are fat-soluble, they stay in the body for a long time, and can severely damage vital organs, including the heart, liver, and kidneys. Repeated use of spray paints can permanently damage the brain and lungs, or cause death by asphyxiation. Sudden sniffing death (SSD) syndrome can happen the first time or any time an inhalant is abused. The heart begins to overwork, beating rapidly but unevenly; this can lead to cardiac arrest (see Heart Attack). Toluene (spray paint) and butane (lighter fluid) are the top causes of SSD.

Because preteens are still growing, the toxic effects of solvents have long-term repercussions on a child's physical, mental, and emotional development. The organ most vulnerable to toxic buildup is the brain (see Brain). Cellular death in the cerebral cortex causes permanent personality changes, impairment of the memory, hallucinations, and learning disabilities.

Substances abused and their hazards		
PRODUCT	**PRINCIPAL CONSTITUENTS**	**MAIN HAZARDS**
Aerosols	Propellants Particles (depending on type of spray)	Damage to lungs Suffocation during direct inhalation
Fire extinguishers	Extinguishant	Accidental death. Heart toxicity.
Impact adhesives and other glues	Solvents Additives	Suffocation, accidental death, brain damage, liver, and kidney damage
Lighter fuel	Fuel gases	Accidental death
Gasoline	Petroleum compounds Additives (including tetraethyl lead)	Accidental death Possible lead poisoning
Correcting fluid	Solvent	Accidental death. Heart toxicity.

Detection, action, and prevention

Signs of solvent abuse are: children may behave as if drunk, their breath may smell of solvents, and the chemicals may cause red nostrils or sores around their mouths. They may appear dreamy and moody, and lose their appetite. Hidden piles of rags, paper or plastic bags, and tubes or cans of glue may confirm that a child has been sniffing solvents. Many deaths result from inhalation of vomit by semiconscious children lying on their back. Someone who is caught abusing solvents must be kept calm or he or she may hallucinate or become violent. The stress can overstimulate the heart, causing palpitations or cardiac arrest. If a person is conscious, he or she must be kept calm in a well-ventilated room. If the person is unconscious or not breathing, an ambulance must be summoned immediately. A person who is unconscious but breathing should be put in the recovery position. If the person is not breathing, mouth-to-mouth ventilation must be done at once. If the person is unresponsive, chest compression can be applied.

Treatment facilities for inhalant users are rare. Chronic users tend to suffer a high rate of relapse, and may require 30 to 40 days of detoxification. Withdrawal symptoms can be as severe as those experienced by alcoholics or heroin addicts. Physical detoxification is followed by individual or group therapy. For all these reasons, prevention is very important. The most effective method of prevention is discussion. Parents and teachers, medical professionals, retailers, elected officials, and law enforcement officers need to be informed of the problem and its dangers. The students often make the best educators, by alerting their peers to the dangers of solvent abuse.

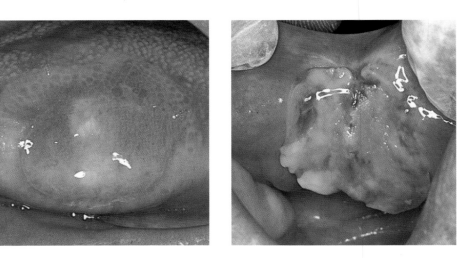

▲ *Apart from the obvious dangers of suffocation, prolonged solvent abuse can cause severe sores in and around the mouth.*

See also: Nervous system

Sores

"Sores" is a general term that describes local damage to the skin resulting from injury, infection, allergy, or some other agency. Treatment may be unnecessary unless a sore persists.

Questions and Answers

Should a sore be covered with a bandage or left uncovered?

It depends on the type of sore. Small, clean open sores should be left uncovered if possible, but it may be more sensible to cover a child's wounded knee to protect it from dirt or to avoid damaging the scab that will form. A dressing or bandage will keep a sore moist, and may slow down healing, so it should not be left on for too long. If there is no obvious infection in the sore do not apply antiseptic ointment; it is better to allow a scab to form.

What is the difference between a sore and an ulcer?

"Sore" is a general lay term covering any kind of skin lesion, such as wounds, ulcers, blisters, and crusts. An ulcer is a specific type of lesion involving loss of tissue, usually, but not always, with inflammation. Ulcers may occur on any surface of the body, external or internal. They may be clean-edged or ragged, shallow or deep, and in some cases may penetrate a tissue wall.

Why do I keep getting cold sores?

Because you were infected with the herpes simplex virus from another person. Cold sores around the lips and mouth take time to heal, and there is no treatment necessary other than petroleum jelly to stop cracking. They recur in people whose resistance to colds is low.

Do acidic foods cause mouth sores?

No. Mouth ulcers occur singly or a few at a time, and have no known cause. They are painful, and eating citrus fruits will cause an ulcer to smart. Mouth sores may be due to dental trouble, so consult a dentist about the problem.

The skin is the body's principal protective covering and it is extremely tough, although it can be injured externally by abrasions, heat and cold, chemicals, and sunlight, and internally by allergic substances, infections, and certain diseases. Any of these agents can produce different injuries or breaks in the skin. A general lay term for a painful, irritating break in the skin is a sore (see Skin and Skin Diseases). Sores develop from many skin conditions. For example, if blisters are broken, the raw patch would be called a sore. Scratching the skin when it is itchy can cause small breaks in the skin which may bleed or become infected.

Cold sores and bedsores

The cold sore is a very common, painful, and irritating condition, usually found around the mouth or nose. It is caused by a virus called herpes simplex (see Herpes). The virus remains in the skin and the cold sore is caused when the sufferer has a cold or resistance is low. No treatment is necessary, since it normally disappears in a few days. Applying petroleum jelly may give relief.

Bedsores are caused by constant, lengthy pressure on the same area of skin, and occur where there is a bone close to the skin. Such areas include the heels, elbows, center of pelvis, and back of the head. Sustained pressure at any of these points compresses the small arteries so that the blood supply to the area is cut off. The result is tissue death, or gangrene. Bedsores develop quickly in unconscious patients, especially those who have taken a narcotic drug overdose, and in people who have had strokes or are immobile because of physical weakness. The most

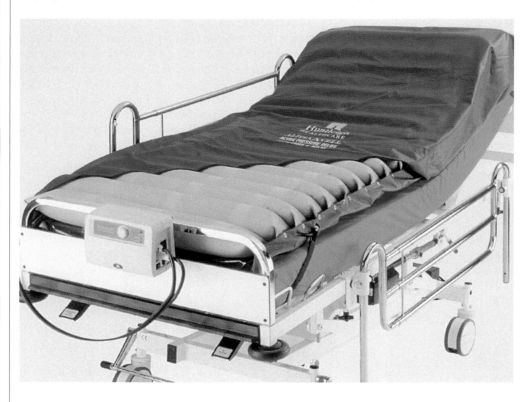

▲ *A patient who is bedridden and unable to move for any length of time may develop bedsores. The computerized active pressure relieving mattress overlay system can help to alleviate this painful condition.*

common site of bedsores is over the sacrum at the base of the spine. Blisters develop which break, and the underlying sore can take a long time to heal. The patient must be turned often and the pressure areas rubbed with a zinc and castor oil cream or surgical spirit to prevent sores. If bedsores do appear, dressings and antibiotics will be necessary for the young; elderly people need nursing.

Genital sores

These have many causes. The sore, which can be caused by intercourse, is painful, is irregular in shape, and may become infected. Syphilis causes a sore, like an ulcer, or chancre. A fungal infection, candidosis (see Thrush), causes sore patches in the vagina and small sores on the foreskin and glans of the penis. Similar sores can be caused in the genital area by sexually transmitted herpes viruses. The herpes virus causes small itchy and painful blisters, which burst and leave small sores. An attack may last for one or two weeks, and often recurs. Herpes genitalis is usually transmitted by sexual contact (see Sexually Transmitted Diseases).

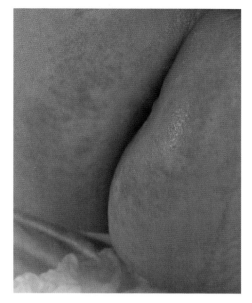

▲ *Those in daily contact with rubber may develop rubber dermatitis.*

▲ *Diaper rash can cause sores caused by bacterial action on the urea in urine.*

Industrial sores

Industrial sores are caused by dust, liquids or vapor, or any other skin irritant in a working environment. About 70 percent of industrial dermatitis is caused by damage to the skin by friction from abrasive dust such as coal, stone, brick, or steel wool. Acids and other chemicals such as paraffin, petroleum, and turpentine can all cause skin damage. After years of exposure of the skin to irritating dusts or liquids, thickening and scaling of the skin often develops. This is common in elderly coal miners or building laborers. Small minor injuries to the skin are slower to heal if the sore is in constant contact with an irritant. People who are exposed to chromic acid and chromates develop ulcers called chrome sores around

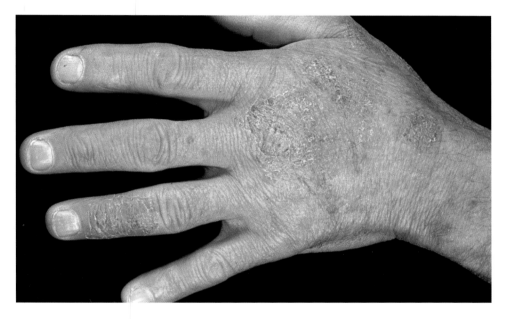

▲ *Those who work with chrome become sensitive after constant exposure to chromic acid and chromates, and risk developing chrome sores.*

cuts and abrasions. These are usually seen on the skin of the fingers and the midline septum of the nose. Another hazard is exposure to radioactive material and X rays that cause acute burns. The burns often develop into sores that are slow to heal. Sometimes a skin cancer may form in the sore.

Tropical sores

Tropical sores are common in the tropics and subtropics and can affect immigrants and visitors. They may also develop in people who have been on vacation in tropical countries. The infection that causes tropical sores is caused by parasites called leishmania. The infection spreads by sandfly bites, which may persist for several weeks. A tropical sore has a shallow break in the center and a scab; after several months an unsightly scar will be left. Some forms of tropical sore may actually destroy the skin and tissues underneath.

Implications of sores

A sore that persists for several weeks should be examined by a doctor. Infection may delay healing, and treatment may be needed. All serious skin conditions benefit from early treatment. The skin should be kept dry; ointments may delay healing. Sores must not be squeezed; this delays healing and causes scars to form.

See also: **Burns; Cancer; Scars**

Sore throat

This common symptom results from inflammation of the throat or the surrounding tissues. In most cases very simple treatment is all that is needed to ease the pain and make a patient more comfortable.

The throat is one of the major passages of the body (see Throat). Air constantly passes up and down from the nose and mouth to the lungs. Food and drink pass through the throat on their way from the mouth to the stomach. Because the throat is the only entry into the lungs or the stomach, all the air that is breathed in and all the food and drink that are taken in have to pass through the throat. The throat is exposed to any material coughed up from the lungs and bronchial passage or vomited up from the stomach.

The tissues that make up and surround the throat (the back of the tongue, the tonsils, the pharynx, and the space at the back of the nose) are constantly exposed to the risk of infection (see Infection and Infectious Diseases), making a sore throat a common human ailment.

Causes

Sore throat is not a disease in itself. The basic feeling of soreness in the throat may be the result of inflammation of any of the surrounding tissues (see Inflammation). In addition, a sore throat is not necessarily caused by one particular germ, since a wide range of bacteria, viruses, and other microorganisms (such as fungi in the case of sore throat due to oral thrush; see Thrush) can attack the throat. In some cases the soreness is due not to infection, but to damage from other sources: swallowing foods and drinks that are too hot, discharge running down from the

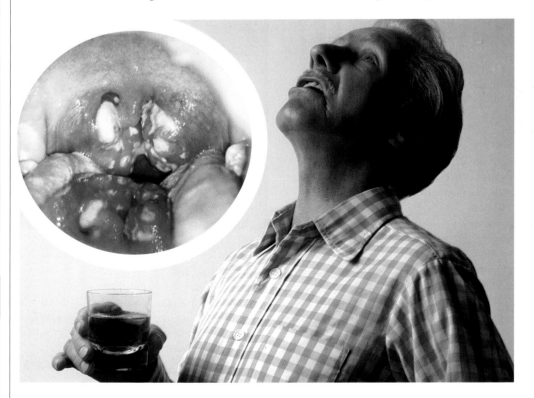

▲ *Gargling, even with something as simple as ordinary salt and water or a mixture of aspirin and water, is an effective way of soothing the symptoms of a sore throat. In a streptococcal throat (inset) the tissues of the throat and neighboring organs have been infected with streptococcus bacteria. This is what the infected area would look like to a doctor examining the patient's throat.*

THROAT AND SURROUNDING TISSUE

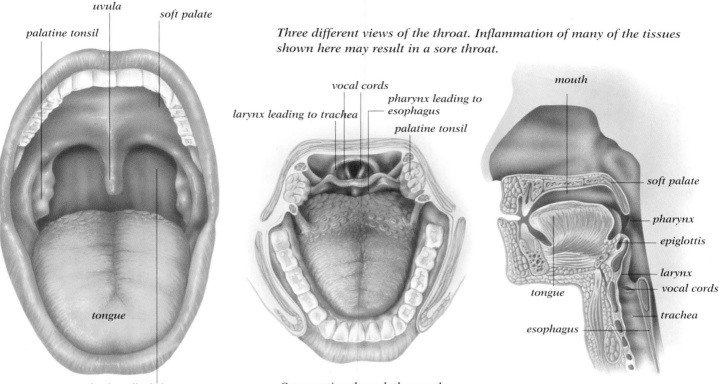

Three different views of the throat. Inflammation of many of the tissues shown here may result in a sore throat.

uvula
soft palate
palatine tonsil

vocal cords
larynx leading to trachea
pharynx leading to esophagus
palatine tonsil

mouth
soft palate
pharynx
epiglottis
larynx
vocal cords
tongue
trachea
esophagus

tongue

back wall of pharynx

Cross section through the mouth

back of the nose (see Nose), excessive smoking (see Smoking), or sucking too many strong sweets.

In some diseases (for example, influenza, scarlet fever, measles, and diphtheria), a sore throat is only the first, and relatively unimportant, symptom of a disease that develops into a condition much more widespread and serious. In most cases of sore throat, however, the trouble is confined to the throat.

The most common cause of sore throat is acute inflammation of the pharynx (see Pharynx), or pharyngitis. Inflammation of the pharynx usually occurs suddenly, with a feeling of dryness, irritation, and soreness. There is a constant desire to clear the throat, pain on swallowing, a persistent dry cough, and often headache and fever. Pharyngitis is usually due to infection by a virus rather than by bacteria, and taking antibiotics not only is ineffective (they do not combat viruses) but may actually make things worse because of unwanted side effects. Like most viral conditions, the infection clears up of its own accord in a few days, and the only worthwhile treatment is to try to relieve the symptoms by means of hot drinks or appropriate gargles, such as aspirin or salt water.

Chronic pharyngitis may be the result of repeated attacks of acute pharyngitis, heavy smoking, working in dust or fumes, infected adenoids or tonsils, or discharge from the back of the nose or sinuses. It is important to find out exactly what is causing the chronic pharyngitis in order to resolve it.

Tonsillitis

Infections which start with a sore throat or pharyngitis often spread to nearby tissues and involve them too. The most commonly affected neighboring organ is the tonsil (see Tonsils). This is likely to

be affected if the sore throat is due to infection with streptococcus bacteria: the septic, or strep, throat. In sore throat associated with tonsillitis the pain becomes more severe and swallowing is almost impossible. The affected tonsils are enlarged and red, the glands are swollen and tender, and the patient develops a high temperature (see Fevers). If the tonsillitis is not treated, quinsy (a peritonsillar abscess) may develop.

Another serious complication of a sore throat occurs when infection spreads from the pharynx upward to the eustachian tube, which leads to the inside of the ear. This causes otitis media, which is characterized by earache as well as a sore throat (see Otitis). Infection may also spread downward from the pharynx into the voice box, or larynx, leading to laryngitis.

Diphtheria, which is much less common than it used to be, is yet another infection that involves a sore throat. This is characterized by the development of a membrane which is dirty gray in color and a sweetish smell to the breath, as well as the sore throat. Diphtheria was once a common cause of death in children and was feared by parents. The germs that cause it secrete a powerful poison, an exotoxin that gets into the bloodstream and is carried to all parts of the body, damaging the heart and other organs. Many children who survived the infection were often left with severely damaged hearts and nervous systems.

The sharp decline in the prevalence of diphtheria has nothing to do with antibiotics; it was the result of almost universal immunization against the disease (see Immunization). Public health authorities in countries in which this is not mandatory are constantly concerned that parents who have never known the disease may become casual about immunization. Regulations in the United States

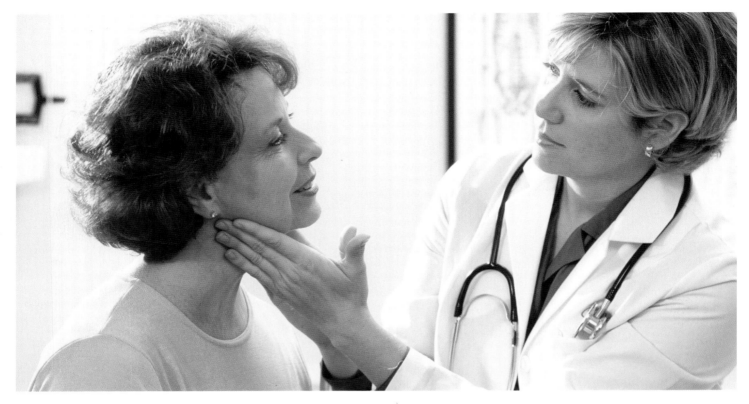

▲ *A doctor examining a sore throat will look down the patient's throat, often with the help of a flashlight, to identify any inflammation that may be present. He or she may also take a throat swab to be sent to a laboratory for identification of the germ involved.*

for schoolchildren make it very unlikely that vaccination levels will drop, but it is important that adults are aware of the danger.

Throat abscess

One of the most acute and alarming complications of tonsillitis is peritonsillar abscess, or quinsy. This starts with a simple sore throat with tonsillitis, which seems to settle down. However, after a few days of comfort the affected person begins to suffer increasing difficulty in swallowing. Pain recurs and usually spreads to the ear on one side. It becomes difficult to open the mouth because of spasm of the chewing muscles, and the speech becomes thick and indistinct. Pain rapidly increases to a level that prevents eating. There is strong pressure in the neck and the head is tilted to the affected side. Rapid head movements are avoided. There is excessive salivation and bad breath. The temperature rises to 101°F (38°C) and the person becomes obviously ill. There may be partial obstruction to the airway by obstruction to the inlet of the voice box (larynx). This will produce difficulty in breathing.

Peritonsillar abscess is caused by a spread of infection from the tonsil to the tissues around and behind it. Occasionally it may arise from an infected and impacted wisdom tooth (third molar). If the inside of the mouth is inspected (which may be difficult because of the difficulty in opening the mouth wide) a distinct, red swelling will be seen, with marked protrusion of the tonsil, on one side.

The uvula (the soft, floppy flap of mucous membrane hanging from the center of the soft palate) is pushed across to the healthy side. The tongue is usually coated and the lymph nodes behind the angle of the jaw on the affected side will be enlarged and tender. Rarely, there may be an abscess on both sides.

Once any abscess, here or elsewhere, is fully developed, antibiotics are useless. This is because the center of an abscess is cut off from the general blood supply and no antibiotics can get to the germs. If severe tonsillitis is treated at an early stage with antibiotics, quinsy will be avoided; and if high-dosage antibiotics are given at an early stage of abscess formation, it may be prevented from becoming established. Painkiller drugs (see Painkillers) are given, an ice pack is applied to the neck, mouthwashes are prescribed, and a cold liquid or semisolid diet is taken. Gargling is useless and, in the presence of partial airway obstruction, dangerous. An established abscess is full of pus (see Pus), and the only effective treatment is to drain the pus through an incision. This is done under local anesthesia and produces an almost immediate and profound relief of pain and other symptoms. In addition to surgery, antibiotics are normally given to cope with the infection that caused the problem.

The surgeon has two options. The first is to open and drain the abscess at the site of maximum protrusion, using a long scalpel which is wrapped in sterile tape so that only the tip is exposed. This is to prevent the danger of injury to the large blood vessels of the neck by too deep penetration. This procedure is followed by removal of the tonsils under general anesthesia (tonsillectomy) three or four days later. Alternatively, tonsillectomy may be done under general anesthesia as the initial procedure. Once the infected tonsils have been removed there is no longer any danger of developing any further quinsies.

Tonsillectomy is almost always done under general anesthesia. The head is tilted back and the mouth is propped open by a ratchet instrument called a gag. Each tonsil in turn is grasped with toothed forceps and is separated from its bed with minimal cutting. This is called blunt dissection. Bleeding from the raw areas left is sometimes brisk, and it is occasionally necessary to secure and close a small bleeding artery by tying it off. In rare cases, severe bleeding occurs some hours after the operation. This will require a return to the operating room for control of the hemorrhage. After tonsillectomy there is severe local discomfort, especially on swallowing, for about two weeks.

Consulting your doctor

Most sore throats are more of a nuisance than an illness, they clear up quickly on their own, and require neither medical advice nor treatment. Nevertheless, some do not clear up, and people should know when it becomes necessary to consult a doctor. If a person has ever had rheumatic fever (see Rheumatic Fever) or nephritis, or a rash develops, or the person is running a fever of 102°F (38.9°C), or if the throat has a gray or yellow coating, he or she may need medical help. He or she should also see a doctor if a sore throat shows no signs of improving by the third day.

The doctor will probably look down the throat with a flashlight. He or she may wipe the back of the throat with a swab and send it to a laboratory for testing, so that the germ that causes the sore throat can be identified and appropriate treatment given. The doctor will also feel the neck for enlarged glands, and examine the nose, ears, and chest to see if they are involved too. If a patient has had a lot of sore throats a doctor may consider it necessary to refer the person to an otolaryngologist for a more conclusive diagnosis.

Self-help

Sore throat is one of those conditions for which people can do a great deal to help themselves. Hot drinks are soothing for a painful throat, and it is worth trying a semisolid food diet so that swallowing is as free from pain as possible. Gargling is also helpful, though probably the relief is due more to the effect of the heat of the gargle than to what is chosen as the gargle. Ordinary salt and water or a mixture of aspirin and water will be effective. A salt gargle can be made simply by putting two teaspoonful of ordinary

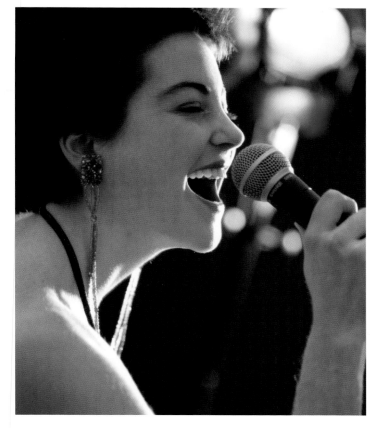

▲ *Singers who use the voice excessively can irritate the larynx to such an extent that the voice is lost and a painful sore throat develops. Rest of the voice is the only treatment.*

household salt in a cup of hot, but not too hot, water and stirring until it is completely dissolved.

Similarly, an aspirin gargle is made by dissolving two soluble aspirin in a cup of hot water. It should be swallowed rather than discarded when gargling is finished so that the aspirin can take effect internally as well by its painkilling and fever-reducing action.

In between gargling it may be helpful to suck a soothing lozenge; fruit pastilles or mentholated lozenges are traditional and effective. If the soreness and irritation in the throat cause coughing, old-fashioned lozenges, sucked as far back in the throat as possible, are safe and soothing. It should be pointed out, however, that the most lozenges will do is soothe a sore throat. Not even the so-called antiseptic lozenges have a specific medicinal property apart from their soothing effect.

▼ **Corynebacterium diphtheriae** *is the organism that causes diphtheria—a potentially fatal infectious disease that is now rarely contracted.*

▼ *The micrograph shows streptococcus bacteria which, by inflaming the tissues of the throat and surrounding organs, often cause sore throats.*

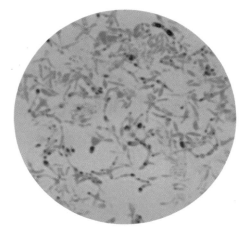

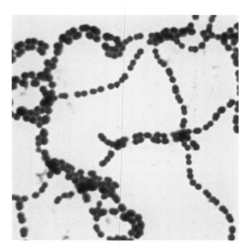

See also: Bacteria; Burns; Diphtheria; Hemorrhage; Influenza; Larynx and laryngitis; Measles; Pain; Scarlet fever; Surgery; Tongue

INDEX

Headings and page numbers in **bold** refer to complete articles. Page numbers in *italics* refer to illustrations or their captions.